Ethnography of Fertility and Birth

Second Edition

Ethnography of Fertility and Birth

Second Edition

Edited by
Carol P. MacCormack

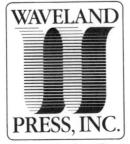

WAVELAND
PRESS, INC.
Prospect Heights, Illinois

For information about this book, write or call:
Waveland Press, Inc.
P.O. Box 400
Prospect Heights, Illinois 60070
(708) 634-0081

Contributors

Sheila Cosminsky
Department of Anthropology, Rutgers University, Camden College of Arts and Sciences, Camden, New Jersey 08102, U.S.A.
Dr. Cosminsky's research in medical and nutritional anthropology includes Belize, Guatemala, Kenya, Zimbabwe and Japan.

Chris Dougherty
Department of Economics, London School of Economics and Political Science, University of London, Houghton Street, London WC2, U.K.
Much of Dr. Dougherty's work in statistics and economics pertains to the field of health economics.

Victoria Ebin
ORSTOM, Equipe du sud, 213 rue Lafayette, Paris 75010, France
Dr. Ebin's work has been with the Organisation pour la Recherche Scientifique en Coopération in Senegal, the Musée de l'Homme in Paris, the Cambridge University Museum and the Brooklyn Museum.

Brenda Gray
Maryland Department of Health and Mental Hygiene, 201 W. Preston Street, Baltimore, Maryland 21201, U.S.A.
Dr. Gray's research in Papua New Guinea and the United States has combined anthropology, epidemiology, health planning and health policy.

Hilary Homans
Overseas Development Administration, P.O. Box 9200, Dar es Salaam, Tanzania
Dr. Homan, a medical sociologist active in the women's health movement, has taught at the University of Zimbabwe and is O.D.A. Health and Population Field Manager for Tanzania.

A. David Jones
39 Blenkarne Road, London SW11 6HZ, U.K.
Dr. Jones was a lecturer in the Department of Social Psychology, London School of Economics and Political Science and is now a psychotherapist in private practice.

Sheila Kitzinger
Standlake Manor near Witney, Oxford OX8 7RH, U.K.
Sheila Kitzinger, MBE, organized the first master's degree programme in midwifery in the U.K., and her books on childbirth are widely read.

Carol MacCormack
Department of Anthropology, Bryn Mawr College, Bryn Mawr, Pennsylvania 19010, U.S.A.
Dr. MacCormack taught at Cambridge and the London School of Hygiene and Tropical Medicine; research includes various anthropological topics and tropical public health.

Dennis McGilvray
Department of Anthropology, University of Colorado, Boulder, Colorado 80309, U.S.A.
Dr. McGilvray's research with matrilineal groups in Sri Lanka encompasses kinship, caste, ethnic relations and the analysis of symbols and ritual.

Una Maclean
Department of Community Medicine, Usher Institute, Warrender Park Road, Edinburgh EH9 1DW, Scotland, U.K.
From her medical background, Dr. Maclean was an early innovator in the modern field of medical anthropology and has given valuable advice to international agencies.

Preface to the Second Edition

In 1979, when Murray Last, at University College London, organized a British Medical Anthropology Society conference on childbirth, he was a bit ahead of his time. Brigitte Jordan's *Birth in Four Cultures* had been published only the year before. (It is now in its fourth edition and destined to be a classic [Jordan, 1993].) The World Health Organization, first in the African Region, then in Geneva, had only recently prepared its first publications on working with traditional midwives to reduce maternal and infant mortality in poor countries with sparse health care coverage (WHO, 1976, 1979). Ethnographic literature that might assist safe motherhood programmes was buried in the periodical literature of anthropology and other social sciences. The first edition of this book grew out of the need for more systematic case studies.

Since 1979, a robust and useful literature has developed. Carol Laderman's study in rural Malaysia (1983), Carolyn Sargent's monographs on birth in Benin (1982, 1989), and Robbie Davis-Floyd's anthropological study of birth in America (1992) are just a few examples. Regrettably, much of the medical and health planning literature ignores detailed studies of culturally appropriate fertility and birth care. The international journal *Social Science and Medicine*, the newsletter of WHO's Safe Motherhood Programme, and a recent book from Uppsala University's Department of Obstetrics and Gynaecology are good examples of medical sensitivity to cultural contexts and economic constraints in poor countries (WHO, 1989; Liljestrand and Povey, 1992). Poor countries have their special constraints and opportunities, and many rich countries suffer from what can only be called a poverty of the spirit in childbirth. These articles remain relevant to the task of informing better fertility and birth care for all women.

References

Davis-Floyd, R. (1992). *Birth as an American Rite of Passage.* Berkeley: University of California Press.

Jordan, B. (1993). *Birth in Four Cultures*, 4th edition. Prospect Heights, Ill.: Waveland Press.

Laderman, C. (1983). *Wives and Midwives: Childirth and Nutrition in Rural Malaysia.* Berkeley: University of California Press.

Liljestrand, J. and Povey, W. G. (eds) (1992). *Maternal Health Care in an International Perspective.* Uppsala: Uppsala University.

Sargent, C. (1982). *The Cultural Context of Therapeutic Choice: Obstetrical Care Decisions Among the Bariba of Benin.* Dordrecht: D. Reidel.

Sargent, C. (1989). *Maternity, Medicine and Power: Reproductive Decisions in Urban Benin.* Berkeley: University of California Press.

World Health Organization (1976). *Training and Supervision of Traditional Birth Attendants.* Brazzavilie: WHO.

World Health Organization (1979). *Traditional Birth Attendants: An Annotated Bibliography of Their Training, Utilization and Evaluation.* Geneva: WHO.

World Health Organization (1989 to present). *Safe Motherhood.* Newsletter of the Safe Motherhood Initiative. Geneva: WHO.

C.P.M.
July 1994

Preface

"Natural Childbirth" and "natural fertility" are phrases that are often used with conviction but with some conceptual imprecision. "Natural fertility" tends to mean the fertility of a population that does not use contraceptive techniques understood in the West. The concept ignores the wide range of cultural rules and social practices which already exist in *every* society to shape the pattern of human fertility. The society has yet to be discovered where humans breed without rules of incest avoidance, marriage, and parental responsibility. Those rules and social behaviours account for our humanity and set us apart from animals who are thought to be governed by biological function only. Nor is human childbirth "natural" in an animal sense, but in all societies it proceeds in a social setting and is given cultural meaning.

Equally in error is an exclusive focus on "birth customs" without an attempt to relate them to the adaptive strategies of a population that is managing to survive in a particular environment. The rules and social procedures of some societies appear more successful in teaching constructive meanings of birth, and in maximizing the reproductive potential of women, than in others.

This book examines that adaptive process in societies ranging from rural agricultural environments to urban industrial settings. The contributors range from physicians to anthropologists, but with considerable overlap in their interests. Most of the papers have been discussed in meetings of the British Medical Anthropology Society, an excellent forum for the melding of biological and socio-cultural perspectives.

C.P.M.
November 1981

ix

Contents

1. Introduction: Biological, Cultural and Social Meanings of Fertility and Birth

C. P. MacCormack

The First and Third Worlds Joined

Do we live in peculiar times? *In vitro* fertilization and other birth technologies are causing us to question the fundamental meaning of kinship. Bombing, burning and shooting at family planning clinics, and court-ordered Caesarean sections have turned the places for fertility and birth care into battle grounds (Strathern, 1992; Handwerker, 1990; Ginsburg, 1989; Whitford and Poland, 1989; Corea, 1985).

If the pursuit of reproductive health in industrial countries sounds like risky business, the average lifetime risk of dying from pregnancy-related causes is about 1 in 15 in some poor countries. By way of contrast, in parts of northern Europe a woman has only a 1 in 10,000 chance of dying in pregnancy and childbirth (Royston and Armstrong, 1989; Jordan, 1993). To put the situation another way, in the world as a whole, every minute a woman dies as a result of complications during pregnancy and birth, and every minute eight babies die because of poor care for their mothers in pregnancy and birth (WHO, 1993). Most deaths, however, occur where there is poverty and women's health needs are neglected. The great tragedy is that between 88 and 98% of maternal deaths could be avoided. A World Health Organization interregional committee concluded that with good access to antenatal care, maternity services for high-risk women, sufficient medical supplies such as blood banks, and adequate training for health workers, those lives could be saved (WHO, 1986). This does not mean expensive technologies or an elaborate hospital infrastructure, but culturally appropriate services at community and district levels (WHO 1993).

1

The complete absence of modern maternity care is a great risk. Maria Lepowsky had described a young woman named Rara, on a remote island off Papua New Guinea, giving birth to her first child. She had been in labour for six days with the foetus probably in a transverse lie position: "the baby's head was still pointing sideways" (1993, p. 81). The island women did not know how to massage the abdomen and attempt an external cephalic version. A life-saving Caesarean section was not a possible option in such a remote place. Several kinswomen supported the young woman, literally sitting behind her to support her lower back with their feet. They gave her kindness and herbal teas. Her father, husband, and a ritual specialist chewed warming ginger root, spraying it upon her stomach and back. They called to the baby to come out: "Come out and we men will go make sago", they sang, inviting the not yet born boy to join them. Another ritual specialist "sucked" an object from Rara's back, declaring it had been obstructing the labour. All looked at the small green object, then it was carried way, far into the forest. Rara's husband chewed root and said magic, addressing the foetus: "I am your father. Hurry up and come out. I want to see you". The fetal position shifted, amniotic fluid flowed, a boy was born and both he and his mother survived. However, Rara was left with reproductive disorders and barrenness for the rest of her life.

This ethnographic observation helps us see how rich and poor countries are linked in a curious way, with Western women having more Caesarian sections than they want or need, and women in poor countries suffering unto death because none are available (Sakala, 1993).

Maternal Mortality

In rural Gambia there is a market town named Farafenni, which in Mandinka means "where the rice fields end". That is another way of saying "the back of beyond". Trucks do come through the area, hoping to cross the River Gambia on an unreliable ferry. The nearest hospital is 200 km away, but The Gambia has one of the best community-based primary health care services in Africa. Nevertheless, maternal mortality in that area in the late 1980s was 2,360 deaths per 100,000 live births (Greenwood *et al.*, 1990). Maternal deaths are only part of the tragedy. For each death about 15 women suffer the physical disability and social ostracism that result from incontinence (bladder and bowel), uterine prolapse, infertility and other consequences of untreated birth trauma (Greenwood *et al.*, 1990). Everywhere in the world the survival chances for children of dead or ostracized women are poor indeed. Those 2,360 maternal deaths contrast with 5 per 100,000 live births in Sweden (WHO, 1991).

A combined rural and urban study in Zimbabwe found that hemorrhage, eclampsia and puerperal sepsis following birth and abortion were the major direct causes of maternal death. In rural areas untreated malaria was the leading indirect cause. Further risk factors were associated with having little social support: being unmarried, divorced, one of several wives, cohabiting outside marriage or being entirely self-supporting. Nearly half of the deaths were women who had pregnancies that were not wanted, and there were four pregnancy-related suicides. Implicit in much of this risk is a huge unmet need for good contraceptive services (Mbizvo *et al.*, 1993).

A comparative study in Ghana, Nigeria and Sierra Leone focused on the interval between the onset of obstetric complications and the birth outcome. Impediments to prompt treatment were distance to a hospital, lack of transportation, cost of transportation and care, and anticipated quality of care. How severe the emergency was and women's social rank also delayed or enhanced the decision to seek help. Once the life-threatened woman reached hospital, shortages of qualified staff and essential drugs, administrative delays and clinical mismanagement were often further impediments to a satisfactory birth (Thaddeus and Maine, 1994).

Pakistan researchers reviewed the cases of 118 pregnant or recently delivered women who were brought dead to Jinnah Hospital in Karachi between 1981 and 1990. All the women were poor and had been looked after by traditional midwives, family members or small maternity homes. Of the 118 women, 48 died of hemorrhage associated with birth or abortion, 25 of eclampsia, 13 of ruptured uterus, and 5 of septicaemia from birth or abortion. Other causes were anaemia and cardiac or liver failure. When family members were asked about delay in bringing the dying woman to hospital, about half the kin replied in terms of economic constraints but a further half spoke of more subtle social and cultural constraints such as the family hesitating to make a decision or the husband not giving approval (Jafarey and Korejo, 1993).

Maternal mortality rates, and also the death rates of girl children compared with boy children, reflect the general social power of women. Countries with some political commitment to social justice and primary health care for all people tend to have lower maternal death rates. For example, China has a maternal mortality rate of 22 per 100,000 live births compared to 833 per 100,000 in Bangladesh (WHO, 1986; MacCormack, 1988). The "green revolution" in north India is often considered a technological and capitalistic success, but it has resulted in less employment for poor women, increased dowry demands for girls in all social classes, increased male dominance as a concomitant of relatively greater employment opportunities for men, and little female education among the poor. As poor girls and women become increasingly marginalized, they seek social status through bearing children. Having many pregnancies is of course a risk factor for maternal mortality. Also, the proportion of female children who do not survive is increasing. Susan Wadley's (1993) interpretation is that poor families in north India are maximizing male survival as insurance against old age and poverty. Among wealthy, land-owning north Indian households some families use genetic screening to abort females and bring to term male foetuses. However, the situation may not be so bad in India as in America. A 19-country survey found that 62% of American medical geneticists would perform antenatal diagnosis to select a male foetus but only 52% of the Indian medical geneticists would help select a male foetus (Wertz and Fletcher, 1993).

Cynthia Myntti gives us insight into further subtle risk factors in her study of Yemen child deaths. Deaths tend to cluster in some families and not in others. Myntti measured mother's age, education, number of children, residential patterns, husband's education and occupation, household sanitation, food hygiene, handwashing, infant feeding, diarrhoea treatment and immunization. Those standard variables did not explain the difference between many deaths in some households and few in others. However, more open-ended anthropological conversations did reveal significant variables. There were few deaths where women were well integrated into social networks of kin, friends and neighbours, and where women had some control over even a meagre household income. Where women had no control and no social support they simply accepted deaths as their fate. Where they did have control and friendship they were often angry and never passive (Myntti, 1993).

Carol Delaney (1991) gives further insight in her excellent interpretation of the rural Turkish world view, which defines procreation as an aspect of divine creation. Divine creation is ultimate, while human procreation is intimate. Between the intimate and the ultimate a whole world is symbolically created. A man's god-like power and authority is based on his power to generate life. He gives life and identity, the seed which sparks life. If one plants barley seed, barley results. Similarly, a man calls into being a child with its particular identity through the seed he plants in his wife's womb, the "field". She is the object; her body is the microcosm of the work of God. A fertile field is defined, fenced or "covered" by ownership. As with land, women must be "covered" under the mantle of a man: father, husband, brother or son. This is symbolized by the headscarf which a woman will not even remove in the final stages of childbirth. Without it a woman would symbolically declare she was "open", genitals on view, open to the advances or attacks of men.

In the rural Turkey of this study most births took place in domestic privacy with female kin and a traditional midwife addressed with respect as "grandmother" assisting. Most Turkish doctors are men and therefore women will not expose themselves. However, Delaney did describe one young woman who gave birth in hospital. She expected that educated doctors would treat her with respect, but the illusion was shattered. She commented, "We are all human, but they treated me as if I was not". Episiotomy was routine but anesthesia was not, even for suturing the cut. Women were screaming and said afterward that was the most painful part of giving birth (Delaney, 1991, pp. 61-62).

Information for Improving Reproductive Health

Much of the international literature on women's reproductive health is based on death rates. As international agencies attempt to mobilize resources and do something about health inequalities, the sheer numbers of women who die in the prime of their lives are effective in winning support. However, as Wendy Graham and Oona Campbell have pointed out, to go the next step the focus must shift from clinical emergency and death to a population-based epidemiological and public health perspective (Graham and Campbell, 1992). Deaths are not just a clinical matter of reproductive pathology but also depend on patterns of risk and prevention, or whether there is a health service providing primary care. This book seeks to extend the discourse wider still to include cultural, social, economic and emotional aspects of risk, prevention and appropriate services.

The ethnographic method used by all contributors to this book combines qualitative and quantitative methods. Very sensitive questions about intimate and honourable aspects of fertility and birth, or sensitive questions about domestic and professional social control strategies, are best approached indirectly. Ethnography is a method developed within anthropology; researchers enter into the daily lives of people being studied. Open-ended conversations allow much more delicate explorations of thought and emotion, and complement the more public, factual information suitable for closed, pre-coded direct questions. Often ethnographers work outside their home cultures in order to view life with more objectivity. But that is not always the case, and two very sensitive chapters in this book were done on home ground (Ch. 9 and Ch. 10).

Ethnographers make very detailed observations of what people say and do. At the analysis and interpretation stages they attempt, as Carol Delaney did in Turkey, to understand the mental template or cultural definitions, values and rules that lie behind observed behaviour. This interpretive process also gives attention to historical pressures that help shape the observations of the moment. What are the legacies of colonialism, the rather hegemonic Western mechanistic medical world view, and the developing country debt and "structural adjustment" packages? Much recent interpretive anthropology has been used to "displace" us from the unexamined assumptions of Western culture so that we can critically reflect back upon it. Robbie Davis-Floyd (1992), for example, has done just that and helps us take a very fresh, critical look at birth as an American rite of passage (see also Marcus and Fischer, 1986).

Ethnographic methods also facilitate cross-cultural comparison so we might begin to have a frame of reference for such questions as what is "natural"? what is humane? or what is reasonable? If episiotomy is rare in The Netherlands and midwife-attended home birth is common, what is the outcome for Dutch women compared with American women (Jordan, 1993)? The following chapters will take up many such questions which lie embedded within the reproductive life cycle.

Health and Life's Cycles

Carol Delaney described a young woman, a bride of six months, being congratulated on her pregnancy. She replied "It is obligatory. My husband and mother-in-law want it; I would have preferred to wait". It was as though she were a spectator to what was taking place inside her (1991, p. 54). We also read of women who desperately want to become pregnant and cannot (McGilvray, Ch. 2; Ebin, Ch. 5; Maclean, Ch. 6; Kitzinger, Ch. 7). Their reasons for wanting to be mothers vary enormously, from culture to culture and from one stage of the life cycle to another. Dennis McGilvray and Victoria Ebin, for example, discuss the meaning of fertility in societies with an ideology of matrilineal descent, and Sheila Kitzinger describes a society where a three-generation matrifocal family structure is common (see also MacCormack and Draper, 1987; Sobo, 1993). Brenda Gray describes a society that is barely replacing itself because of the interaction of poor nutrition, chronic infection, physical demands of menstruation, pregnancy and lactation and heavy daily farming and domestic work which are heaped upon women, depleting them and bringing them early to old age (Ch. 3).

Everywhere "natural" fertility is shaped by cultural rules. In some cultures family honour, and perhaps dowry or bridewealth as well, are maximized by very early age of marriage for girls. Elders gain in the same process that heightens maternal mortality risk for girls barely in their teens. If a "good" marriage is culturally defined as monogamous, does the culture allow or even encourage extra-marital sexuality to one or both partners? If it is polyandrous, the procreative ability of a set of husbands is limited by the fertility of their one wife. With polygyny, a husband visits his wives occasionally. This reduces fertility for some or all wives who are not visited often because coitus is not sure to take place at the right time in their ovulatory cycle. If women marry at puberty, and men marry first and subsequent wives ten and more years later, as is common with polygyny, will fecund widows be encouraged to remarry or should they remain celibate? If divorce is allowed, women may spend long periods without a partner. Husbands may be away for long periods as herders, traders, fishermen, soldiers, or taking their leisure in men's houses.

Especially in poor countries, few women expect help with their infertility from biomedically trained doctors, and they therefore turn to the traditional sector (Ebin, Ch.5; Maclean, Ch. 6). Some cultural rules and patterns have a secondary effect of putting populations more at risk to fertility-destroying sexually transmitted diseases, or life-destroying conditions such as AIDS. The use and mis-use of indigenous and Western contraceptives and abortifacients also fits within cultural contexts (see for example Lepowsky, 1993, pp. 84–85; Van der Geest and Whyte, 1991; Bamgboye and Lapido, 1992). Even good national health service contraceptives may become conceptually caught up in political and ethnic rivalry and become locally suspect (McGilvray, Ch. 2).

Several contributors have written about the relationship between female body fat and fertility. Where women's proportion of fat compared with lean body weight drops below 20 to 22%, they cease to ovulate. This appears to be an adaptive physiological protection against women falling pregnant in the midst of famine (Frisch, 1988). Some societies also have cultural rules and rituals that require energy-dense foods at puberty and the time of marriage, to maximize plumpness—often synonymous with beauty—and early fecundity (McGilvray, Ch. 2; MacCormack, Ch. 4; Ebin, Ch. 5). Other societies encourage a very meagre diet and girls may take as much as half their average life span to become fecund (Gray, Ch. 3). Cultural rules may also encourage prolonged breastfeeding and frequent suckling, which have the double effect of keeping lactating women's proportion of body fat low and their ovulation-inhibiting prolactin levels high (McGilvray, Ch. 2; Gray, Ch. 3;, MacCormack, Ch. 4; Maclean, Ch. 6). There may be very explicit rules forbidding a woman to resume sexual relations while breastfeeding and the child may remain at the breast for two or more years in environments without energy-dense soft weaning foods (Howell, 1979). Beliefs are widespread throughout the world that semen and breastmilk can mingle in the mother causing harm to the weaned child.

For all the above reasons, we should view the concept of "natural fertility" as our Western cultural construct about others, and abandon the concept in favour of detailed studies of the ways in which particular societies manage fertility. Only then will we be able to offer the kind of culturally appropriate family planning assistance that meets the needs of women and the planet we all share.

Once a woman becomes pregnant the social support she can expect is often dependent on other aspects of social organization. In industrial societies with neolocal residence, husbands or partners, together with hospital or clinic staff, are most likely to look after a woman through pregnancy and birth (Homans, Ch. 9; Jones and Dougherty, Ch. 10). Where marriages tend to be unstable, women often give birth in their mothers' homes or in impersonal institutions (Kitzinger, Ch. 8; Jones and Dougherty, Ch. 10). If there is an ideology of matrilineal descent and matrilocal residence following marriage, a woman in labour is attended by her mother and female kin. Because her fertility directly ensures the continuity of the lineage, she is usually very well cared for by them (McGilvray, Ch. 2).

Where patrilineal descent and patrilocal residence following marriage are the cultural rule, a bride often goes to live among strangers under the authority of her mother-in-law. The mother-in-law is proxy for the men of the lineage who rely on the in-marrying wife to provide lineage continuity. However, young wives often feel very isolated and vulnerable, and they probably have better birth outcomes where they are allowed to return to the safe care of their mothers. The patrilineal-type of societies, with rules of domestic seclusion for women, usually are least likely to have good primary health care services which include female health workers who might assist women where they live.

Once labour begins, few women are entirely on their own. Carolyn Sargent has described the way a Bariba woman in Benin may leave the women assisting her, go into another room, and give birth alone to demonstrate how strong she is (1982, 1989). But the birthing woman is not entirely on her own, and others rush to her assistance if necessary. Only among sparse populations of hunters and gatherers or nomads do we have accounts of women sometimes giving birth without any assistance at all (Shostak, 1983).

In sparsely-populated societies there may not be any woman who can be identified as a traditional midwife (Scheepers, 1991; Alto et al., 1991). Among settled agricultural people, however, traditional midwives are common. In the Indian sub-continent they tend to be of low caste and low status, the people who deal with pollution (McGilvray, Ch. 2; Jeffery *et al.*, 1988). In most of the rest of the world traditional midwives are respected women who may have considerable religious, social and political influence, and provide a range of practical services (MacCormack, Ch. 4; Kitzinger, Ch. 7; Cosminsky, Ch. 8). A primary health care system that does not include all those valuable women who are already providing health services, have a traditional legitimacy to heal, and are keen to enhance their status by learning new skills, is squandering a precious human resource as well as provoking political factionalism at the local level (MacCormack, 1981; Cham *et al.*, 1987). Health planners who dream of mature traditional midwives all being replaced by young women with schoolbook certificates are not connected with the real world of the meaning of birth. Nor are they aware of the real constraints of cost, lack of transportation and "fear of disrespectful or painful treatment from medical personnel" which keep women away from the "modern" health sector (Eades *et al.*, 1993; see also Last and Chavunduka, 1986). However, if traditional midwives, who do far more than the demeaning term "traditional birth attendant" implies, are to have enhanced skills, then training programmes must approach them with respect and share significant practical skills with them (Jordan, 1989).

Nowhere in the ethnographic literature is there a description of women giving birth flat on their backs; traditional midwives, who are themselves mothers, are too wise to propose such a posture. Labouring women walk about, eat, drink, gossip, joke, until they feel they want to squat, sit or lean. They are usually physically supported by other people (see for example Galba-Araujo, 1980). Traditional midwives, facing the labouring woman, may use their feet to support the perineum (MacCormack, Ch. 4), to assist in widening the pelvic outlet (Barns, 1980, p. 315), or use their hands to massage abdomen and perineum to both relax and extend muscles (Cosminsky, Ch. 8).

Among poor women everywhere anaemia is a huge risk factor in childbirth (Royston and Armstrong, 1989). In this review of literature from Vietnam, northern Thailand, Burma, India, east and west Africa, Jamaica, Mexico, Guatemala and Brazil, all descriptions are of the umbilical cord being cut after the placenta is expelled (Mathews and Manderson, 1980, p. 5; Mougne, 1979, p. 77; Philpott, 1980, p. 336; Barns, 1980, p. 316; Swantz, 1969, p. 69; WHO Brazzaville, 1976, p. 124; Kitzinger, Ch. 4; Jordan, 1993, p. 40; Cosminsky, Ch. 7; Galba-Arauja, 1980, p. 295). Training manuals for traditional midwives teach standard industrial society hospital orthodoxy of cutting the cord quickly after the baby is born. Only the sensitive manual by Maureen Williams says "every drop of blood the baby gets from its mother is worth having. If cutting the cord after the

placenta is expelled is the local tradition, it is well worth encouraging''
(1980, p. 27). Neonatal tetanus can be avoided by cauterizing the severed
umbilical cord (Cosminsky, 1978), sterilizing with local gin, or using other
easily available resources.

In the post-partum period massage, steaming baths and other practices
give comfort, restore muscle tone and may promote lactation, creating
''milk kinship'' between mother and child (Kitzinger, Ch. 7; Cosminsky,
Ch. 8; Maher, 1992). Throughout the world, pregnancy is seen as a ''hot''
condition and the post-partum period is a rapid plunge into ''coldness'',
which must be balanced by foods in the right category, warming fires and
other nurturing protections. In a physiological sense, birth is the liminal
stage between two radically different hormonal states, and this sheltered
post-partum care must surely be physically, emotionally and spiritually
good for all who are making those rapid adjustments.

Conclusion

In stark contrast to medical literature, the ethnographic literature locates
fertility and birth within cosmological, social, psychological and spiritual
contexts. Sheila Kitzinger vividly describes how the same spiritual resources
are called upon in ecstatic religious experience and birth. Are the women
who call on those resources ''animals'' as health professionals believe (Ch.
7)? Puberty rites and birth are prime rites of passage, often conceptually
linked, vivid with symbolic expression of women's reproductive power
(McGilvray, Ch. 2; MacCormack, Ch. 4; Kitzinger, Ch. 7; Homans, Ch.
9). Infertility, the other side of birth, is also rich with symbolic meanings,
a time to harmonize people within social and spiritual systems (Ebin, Ch.
5). Robbie Davis-Floyd (1992) has done an excellent job of analyzing the
symbolic statements of hospital birth in an industrial society rite of passage.
How much of that medical model should be exported as ''culturally tied
aid'' to non-Western societies? Hilary Homans (Ch. 9) reminds us that
such rites reproduce the values held by politically dominant groups and
encourage a particular sexual and social division of labour.

A. David Jones and Chris Dougherty (Ch. 10) give us valuable insight
into industrial societies that devalue mothering roles and cause many women
to confront birth neither conceptually nor emotionally prepared for the
changes a rite of passage brings. Women lacking a strong sense of personal
identity and social worth may find the liminal stage in hospital an unbearable
process of depersonalization. They are also apprehensive about the postpartum stage of ''aggregation'' back into society with a new social status

and its accompanying implications—the loneliness and boredom of mothering in isolated nuclear families (see also Homans, Ch. 9). At the very time a woman needs emotional resources to re-think mothering in terms of her relationship with her own mother, and to re-negotiate an emotional relationship with her husband or partner, she is depleted. The destructive effects on her emotions are even greater if the baby is physically defective or dead. All—mother and hospital staff alike—feel themselves "failures". We begin to understand why staff resort to routinization, secrecy and depersonalization to keep from being overwhelmed. It is a world apart from the slow pace, jokes, gossip, and cat naps of village women upholding their neighbour and kinswoman on her heroic journey toward motherhood.

References

Alto, W., Albu, R. and Irabo, G. (1991). "An Alternative to Unattended Delivery: A Training Programme for Village Midwives in Papua New Guinea." *Social Science and Medicine* **32**, 613–618.

Bamgboye, E. and Lapido, O. (1992). "Oral Contraceptive Marketing in Ibaden, Nigeria". *Social Science and Medicine* **35**, 903–906.

Barns, T. (1980). "The Indigenous Midwife in India". In *Maternity Services in the Developing World*. Proceedings of the Seventh Study Group of the Royal College of Obstetrics and Gynaecologists (R. H. Philpott, ed.), pp. 311–322.

Cham, K., MacCormack, C., Touray, A. and Baldeh, S. (1987). "Social Organization and Political Factionalism: Primary Health Care in The Gambia". *Health Policy and Planning* **2**, 214–226.

Corea, G. (1985). *The Mother Machine: Reproductive Technologies from Artificial Insemination to Artificial Wombs*. New York: Harper and Row.

Cosminsky, S. (1978). "Midwifery and Medical Anthropology". In *Modern Medicine and Medical Anthropology in the United States-Mexico Border Population* (B. Velimirovic, ed.), pp. 116–126. Washington, D.C.: Pan American Health Organization.

Davis-Floyd, R. (1992). *Birth as An American Rite of Passage*. Berkeley: University of California Press.

Delaney, C. (1991). *The Seed and the Soil: Gender and Cosmology in Turkish Village Society*. Berkeley: University of California Press.

Eades, C., Brace, C., Osei, L. and LaGuardia, K. (1993). "Traditional Birth Attendants and Maternal Mortality in Ghana". *Social Science and Medicine* **36**, 1503–1507.

Frisch, R. (1988). "Fatness and Fertility". *Scientific American* **258**, 88–94.

Galba-Araujo, A. (1980). "The Traditional Birth Attendant in Brazil". In *Maternity Services in the Developing World* (R. H. Philpott, ed.), pp. 293–310. Proceedings of the Seventh Study Group of the Royal College of Obstetricians and Gynaecologists, London.

Ginsburg, F. (1989). *Contested Lives: The Abortion Debate in an American Community*. Berkeley: University of California Press.

Graham, W. and Campbell, O. (1992). "Maternal Health and the Measurement Trap". *Social Science and Medicine* 35, 967–977.

Greenwood, A., Bradley, A., Byass, P., Greenwood, B., Snow, R., Bennett, S. and Hatib-N'Jai, A. (1990). "Evaluation of a Primary Health Care Programme in The Gambia: The Impact of Trained Traditional Birth Attendants on the Outcome of Pregnancy". *Journal of Tropical Medicine and Hygiene* 93, 58–66.

Handwerker, W. P. (ed.) (1990). *Births and Power: Social Change and the Politics of Reproduction*. Boulder: Westview Press.

Howell, N. (1979). *Demography of the Dobe !Kung*. New York: Academic Press.

Jafarey, S. and Korejo, R. (1993). "Mothers Brought Dead: An Enquiry into Causes of Delay". *Social Science and Medicine* 36, 371–372.

Jeffery, P., Jeffery, R. and Lyons, A. (1988). *Labour Pains and Labour Power*. London: Zed Press.

Jordan, B. (1989). "Cosmopolitical Obstetrics: Some Insights from the Training of Traditional Midwives". *Social Science and Medicine* 28, 925–944.

Jordan, B. (1993). *Birth in Four Cultures*, 4th edition. Prospect Heights, Ill.: Waveland Press.

Last, M. and Chavunduka, G. (eds) (1986). *The Professionalisation of African Medicine*. Manchester: Manchester University Press.

Lepowsky, M. (1993). *Fruit of the Motherland: Gender in an Egalitarian Society*. New York: Columbia University Press.

MacCormack, C. (1981). "Health Care and the Concept of Legitimacy". *Social Science and Medicine* 15B, 423–428.

MacCormack, C. (1988). "Health and the Social Power of Women". *Social Science and Medicine* 26, 677–684.

MacCormack, C. and Draper, A. (1978). "Social and Cognitive Aspects of Female Sexuality in Jamaica". In *The Cultural Construction of Sexuality* (P. Caplan, ed.), pp. 143–165. London: Tavistock.

Maher, V. (ed.) (1992). *The Anthropology of Breastfeeding: Natural Law or Social Construct?* Oxford: Berg.

Marcus, G. and Fischer, M. (1986). *Anthropology as Cultural Critique*. Chicago: University of Chicago Press.

Mathews, M. and Manderson, L. (1980). "Vietnamese Behavioural and Dietary Precautions During Confinement". Department of Indonesian and Malayan Studies, University of Sidney.

Mbizvo, M., Fawcus, S., Lindmark, G. and Nystrom, L. (1993). "Maternal Mortality in Rural and Urban Zimbabwe: Social and Reproductive Factors in an Incident Case-Referent Study". *Social Science and Medicine* 36, 1197–1205.

Mougne, C. (1979). "Changing Patterns of Fertility in a North Thai Village". Paper presented to the Australian Anthropological Society, University of Sidney.

Myntti, C. (1993). "Social Determinants of Child Health in Yemen". *Social Science and Medicine* 37, 233–240.

Philpott, R. H. (ed.) (1980). *Maternity Services in the Developing World*. Proceedings of the Seventh Study Group of the Royal College of Obstetricians and Gynaecologists, London.

Royston, E. and Armstrong, S. (eds) (1989). *Preventing Maternal Deaths*. Geneva: World Health Organization.

Sakala, C. (ed.) (1993). Special Issue of *Social Science and Medicine* on "Caesarean Section Birth in the U.S." **37**, 1177–1281.

Sargent, C. (1982). *The Cultural Context of Therapeutic Choice: Obstetrical Care Decisions Among the Bariba of Benin*. Dordrecht: D. Reidel.

Sargent, C. (1989). *Maternity, Medicine and Power: Reproductive Decisions in Urban Benin*. Berkeley: University of California Press.

Scheepers, L. (1991). "Jidda: The Traditional Midwife of Yemen?" *Social Science and Medicine* **33**, 959–962.

Shostak, M. (1983). *Nisa: The Life and Words of a !Kung Woman*. New York: Vintage.

Sobo, E. (1993). *One Blood: The Jamaican Body*. Albany: State University of New York Press.

Strathern, M. (1992). *Reproducing the Future: Anthropology, Kinship and the New Reproductive Technology*. London: Routledge.

Swantz, M. L. (1969). *Religious and Magical Rites of Bantu Women in Tanzania*. Thesis, University of Dar es Salaam.

Thaddeus, S. and Maine, D. (1994). "Too Far to Walk: Maternal Mortality in Context". *Social Science and Medicine* **38**, 1091–1110.

Van der Geest, S. and Reynolds Whyte, S. (eds) (1991). *The Context of Medicines in Developing Countries*. Amsterdam: Het Spinhuis.

Wadley, S. (1993). "Family Composition Strategies in Rural North India". *Social Science and Medicine* **37**, 1367–1376.

Wertz, D. and Fletcher, J. (1993). "Prenatal Diagnosis and Sex Selection in 19 Nations". *Social Science and Medicine* **37**, 1359–1366.

Whitford, L. and Poland, M. (eds) (1989). *New Approaches to Human Reproduction*. Boulder: Westview Press.

Williams, M. (1980). *The Training of Traditional Birth Attendants: Guidelines for Midwives Working in Underdeveloped Countries*. London: Catholic Institute for International Relations.

World Health Organization (1976). *Training and Supervision of Traditional Birth Attendants*. Brazzaville: Regional Office for Africa, WHO.

World Health Organization (1986). "Maternal Mortality: Helping Women Off the Road to Death". *WHO Chronicle* **40**, 175–183.

World Health Organization (1991). Maternal Mortality Ratios Rates: A Tabulation of Available Information, 3rd edition. Geneva: WHO.

World Health Organization (1993). *Progress Report 1991–1992*. Geneva: Maternal Health and Safe Motherhood Programme, WHO.

2. Sexual Power and Fertility in Sri Lanka: Batticaloa Tamils and Moors

D. B. McGilvray

Introduction

Ritual and Medicine

Recent research in South Asia has begun to explore the connections between formal systems of traditional medicine and the colourful, often varied, patterns of public and domestic ritual. Some of the results have been quite promising, demonstrating that ideas of ritual temperature, configurations of colour, states of pollution and possession, and the attributes of male versus female sexuality are often linked by an implicit ritual logic which has wide distribution in South Asia (Beck, 1969; Babb, 1975). While indigenous systems of formal medicine, particularly Ayurvedic theory, continue to exert strong influence on popular ideas of health and disease, there also seem to be significant degrees of regional and cultural variation in the way these orthodox medical traditions are interpreted (Obeyesekere, 1976). The alleviation of suffering and the promotion of health in South Asia generally involve recourse to both medicine and ritual, and the two are therefore intricately linked by compatible logics. In this paper I present information regarding indigenous understanding of the human reproductive process within a distinctive matrilineal Hindu and Muslim region of Sri Lanka. The results suggest some of the ways in which both traditional Ayurvedic medicine and the broad logic of South Asian ritual process may be integrated with variant cultural beliefs and social organization.

A Multi-Ethnic Matrilineal Society

In the regional geography of Sri Lanka, the east coast Tamil speaking Hindu and Muslim settlements extending north and south of the town of Batticaloa are recognized as sharing a number of distinctive cultural and social structural features not found in the Sinhalese Buddhist highlands (Yalman, 1967), the south-western low country (Obeyesekere, 1967), the central dry zone (Leach, 1961), or even the northern Tamil Hindu peninsula of Jaffna (Banks, 1957; David, 1973). The Batticaloa region shares a distinctive dialect of Tamil, reflecting its physical isolation, its ecological unity, and its own historical roots, but the most strikingly different things about Batticaloa are reflected in its social structure and its cultural traditions. Leaving aside the Sinhalese Buddhist colonists who occupy new lands to the west, and the local concentrations of Christians in some of the towns, the population of the Batticaloa region is divided more or less evenly between the Tamils, who are Saivite Hindus, and the Moors, who are Sunni (Shāfi) Muslims. Both of these groups speak the Tamil language and live in adjacent, densely populated, but ethnically segregated, villages and semi-urban wards. Although there are some fishing villages, the majority of the population live by cultivating wet-rice on tracts of land located inland to the west, across the many lagoons which penetrate the region. The data presented in this paper were gathered primarily in the multi-ethnic town of Akkaraipattu (population 25 000, in Amparai District) and in the rural vicinity of Kokkatticcolai (in Batticaloa District), the latter being typical of the dispersed, mainly Hindu, villages and hamlets situated farther inland (see also McGilvray, 1973, 1974, and in press).

The Hindu Tamils of Batticaloa are divided among major castes ranging from Mukkuvar and Vēḷālar Cultivators and Vīracaiva Kurukkaḷ Priests at the top end of the hierarchy, through Fishermen, Smiths and Toddy-tappers in the middle, to Barbers, Washermen and Paraiyar Funeral Drummers at the bottom. The most unusual features of this caste system are the principles of matrilineal caste affiliation, the sanctioned intermarriage between some high castes in some localities, and the existence of a traditional Vīracaiva (Lingāyat) sectarian priesthood instead of the usual Hindu Brahman caste ritual experts and pandits. Kinship for the Tamils and the Moors follows the Dravidian structure discussed by Yalman (1967), which features a bilateral cross-cousin marriage preference. Within each Tamil caste, and within the Moorish community as a whole, one finds a number of dispersed exogamous matrilineal clans (kuṭi) which have an important role to play in the management of Hindu temples and Muslim mosques. Marriage throughout the region is based on a matri-uxorilocal residence pattern in which, following a wedding in the bride's house, the married couple continue to reside with the bride's parents and unmarried siblings. Later, the married daughter takes full possession of the natal house in fulfilment of her dowry, while her parents and some or all of her unmarried siblings move to another house nearby. Today inheritance is chiefly channelled through the daughters' dowry, and sons await the usufruct of the property their own brides will bring in marriage. Although matrilineal organization in the Batticaloa region lacks the corporate solidarity of the classic joint matrilineal households (*taravād*) of Kerala, there is widespread recognition of the principle of matriliny (*tāy vali*, "mother-way") and of the special importance of maternal relations. This is not merely fortuitous, for the social structure of the Batticaloa region has historical connections with the society of the Malabar Coast.

Indigenous Medical Theory

Although the Batticaloa region as a whole preserves many distinctive cultural traditions, the spread of Western science and medicine, the availability of books and periodicals published in Colombo, Jaffna and Madras, and the growing sense of cultural unity within the larger Tamil speaking world of Sri Lanka and south India all exert increasing influence upon popular thinking in the realms of politics, religion, and traditional medicine. While Batticaloa is a "matrilineal non-Brahman" culture area, the rest of Tamil speaking Sri Lanka, as well as practically all of Tamil Nadu in south India, is patrilineal in emphasis, giving greater salience to Brahmanical orthodoxy in ritual and belief. It was not surprising, then, that people with whom I spoke occasionally found themselves in a conceptual muddle when it came to explaining the role of paternal versus maternal elements, or reconciling Ayurvedic and Western medical theories, in discussions of conception and childbirth. Nevertheless, consensus was quite strong on most points, and a picture of ethnophysiological belief in Batticaloa can now be presented. This information was elicited from a wide range of people, both Hindu and Muslim, but the largest number were local non-Western curing specialists who practise a variant of the Ayurvedic medical system.[1]

At the outset it should be mentioned that people in Batticaloa uniformly classify traditional and modern knowledge about the functioning of the body and the treatment of somatic disorders through the manipulation of daily regimen and diet, and the application of curative

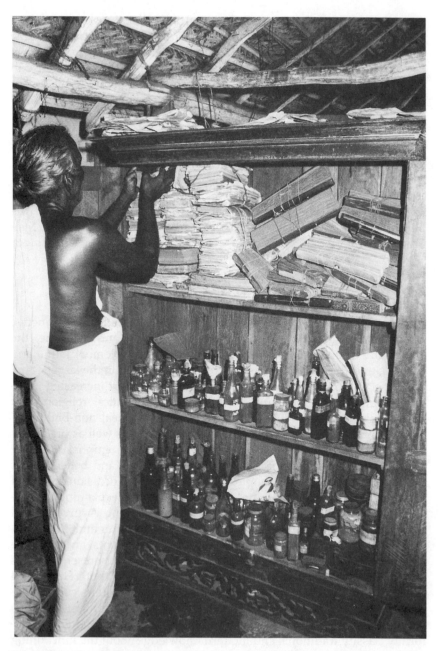

Fig. 1. The office of a Tamil Ayurvedic physician in Tambiluvil, eastern Sri Lanka. Some traditional palm-leaf medical books are piled on the upper right-hand shelf, while his own herbal compounds and oils are stored below.

substances, under the general heading of *vaittiyam*, which corresponds quite closely to our Western category of "medical knowledge". The local belief system, however, is pluralistic, accommodating several other systems of etiology of illness, including astrological influences, the curse or blessing of particular gods and goddesses, the intercession of Muslim saints, and the use of various techniques of sorcery which typically entail possession by one or more low, but extremely malevolent, demons. The fundamental processes of human reproduction are subsumed under *vaittiyam*, medical knowledge, but supernatural influences of various sorts may impinge to disrupt these natural processes. There is no division between Hindu and Muslim folk medicine, although supernatural beliefs are somewhat different.[2]

Blood and Humoural Balance

Blood, which in some parts of South Asia is reported to have extremely important symbolic associations as the locus of caste purity and caste rank, is seen in Batticaloa as the immediate source of health and vitality but is conceptually disjunct from questions of caste. *Irattam onṟu tāṉ*, "blood is all the same", I was told. If different castes had different kinds of blood, said one man, each group would have to receive separate kinds of medication for identical symptoms. The rank and privileges of the different clans, castes and communities in this region are quite clearly marked, but they do not receive conceptual validation in terms of the "purity of caste blood".[3] However, blood (*irattam, utaram*) is definitely recognized to be the primary transformation of food within the body, the source of all bodily substance and strength. An idealized digestive process was often outlined to me as follows: food, which in Sri Lanka is epitomized by boiled rice, is taken into the alimentary tract and converted to *aṉṉaracam* or chyme, which in turn is separated into waste (*malam*) and blood. It is the strength and quantity of the blood which accounts for the strength (*pelaṉ, cakti*) and growth (*vaḷarcci*) of the body. The English word "force" (*pōs*) has crept into the local Tamil vocabulary, and it is sometimes used in describing the condition of the blood. In this context, the term *pōs* evokes at once the vitality, the volume and the hydraulic pressure of the blood in the arterial system. The process of physiological maturation from infancy to adulthood is seen as a direct consequence of the increasing "force" of the blood in the body, and the process of aging and senescence is likewise believed to be a result of an overall decline in the condition of the blood.[4] "My blood has dwindled away" (colloquially, *irattam kuṟaiñci pōyṭṭu*), remarked my elderly Tamil landlord one morning when his rheumatism was acting up. The blood may be weakened in many other ways: it may be thinned-out, mixed with impurities, or (despite the fact that blood is always intrinsically "hot") it may become overheated, resulting in a condition called *irattakkotippu*, "boiling-over of the blood". In fact, despite the reduction of their blood, the elderly do not necessarily "cool off" (see the section on "Contraception: Traditional and Modern" below).

The nature of one's diet, the features of one's environment and the elements of one's daily regimen all have effects upon the internal state of the body, and all these factors are related, with varying degrees of sophistication by different informants, to the influence of the three Ayurvedic humours (*muppini*): namely, *vātam* or *vāyvu* (wind, the source of motion), *pittam* (bile, the source of heat) and *cilērpaṇam* or *cilēṭṭumam* (phlegm, the connective or aqueous humour). Professional Ayurvedic physicians are capable of recognizing extremely subtle and complex combinations of humoural influences, but for most ordinary people in Batticaloa, there is paramount concern for environments, substances and foods conveying the three following qualities: *cūṭu* (heating), *kuḷir* (cooling) and *kiranti* (eruptive). These qualities do not necessarily co-incide with physical properties (e.g. ice is considered to be "heating"), and technically *kiranti* may be a variant of *cūṭu*. However, these are the categories of everyday household concern, and more elaborate di-agnosis is referred to the local specialists. As one might expect, the ideal of bodily health is an equilibrium of these qualities: not too much heat, not too much coolness, not too much eruptive quality. When an imbalance is detected, compensations are made in diet and regimen.

The "heating" and "eruptive" qualities so strongly associated with specific substances and physical conditions can also be engendered in the body through supernatural agency, especially through the anger and displeasure of those fierce female deities so commonly associated in South Asian religion with disease and drought. The cult of such goddesses (Māriyammaṉ, Pattirakāḷi, Turōpatai and Kaṉṉaki being the chief local deities, while lesser known goddesses may be worshipped in domestic rituals) emphasizes their anger and heat, and it is a major objective of the calendrical festivals to pacify and cool them. A very severe outbreak of dermatological pustules or eruptions of any kind, particularly if it occurs on the head or face, is usually taken as the "sign" (*kuṟi*) of an angry goddess' physical presence in the body of the patient. At that stage, application of any cooling substance except mar-gosa leaf is futile and possible insulting to the goddess; there is little one can do but reverently wait for *ammāḷ* (a generic "mother goddess" epithet) literally to "climb down" (*iraṅku*) from the head of the patient.

There is a connection, demonstrated for other parts of South Asia by Beck (1969) and Babb (1975), between the imagery of such ferocious goddesses and the popularly received understanding of unmarried (hence unconstrained) womanhood. At the most abstract metaphysical level, Hindu thought links the male principle with coolness, form and trancendence, while the female principle is linked to heat, energy (*cakti*) and worldly action. The male and female aspects of the universe should theoretically operate as a balanced unity, but there is nevertheless a widespread androcentric preoccupation in South Asia with containing and controlling female energy. This theme is reflected in what my Batticaloa friends said about adolescence and sexual maturity.

The Control of Sexuality

As a child grows toward adulthood, its intake of food sustains the steady production of blood, from which all other bodily substances are produced. But as the body approaches its adult size and form, the body no longer needs to convert so much blood into flesh and bone, and consequently a surplus of blood starts to become available. It is at this point that sexual maturation occurs. Puberty is more dramatic and sudden in the case of girls, because, according to local belief, females produce more blood than males. This fits with the metaphysical notion of *cakti*, energy associated with females, since blood is the locus of bodily energy par excellence. The onset of a girl's first menstruation is both a result of, and a proof of, the fact that her body now has excess or waste blood (*kaḷivirattam*) to dispose of. One view is that her "blood sac" (*irattappai*) gradually fills and then spills out at menstruation. Not all informants were able to offer a cogent explanation of the menstrual cycle, but there was considerable agreement that, without it, women would have dangerously high levels of blood in their bodies, much higher than those of men. The monthly flow of menstrual blood is said to be a safeguard, instituted by Lord Civa, insuring that a woman's natural surplus of blood (and hence physical strength and vitality, including sexual desire) is regularly drained away, allowing men to retain control over women. One local Hindu Ayurvedic practitioner asserted to me: "If it were not for her monthly period, five men could not hold one woman down!"

Blood is also the source of the sexual fluids: hence, it is only when a person reaches puberty, and excess blood is being produced, that sexual feelings are believed to arise. Pre-pubertal children of both sexes are considered to be intrinsically pure of body and mind, and they are often given special roles to play in Hindu ritual because of this. Boys

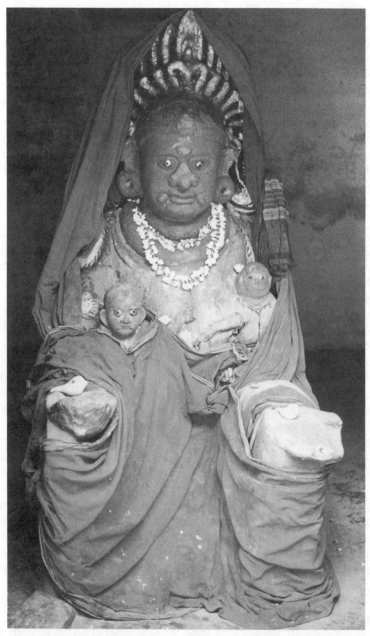

Fig. 2.   Image of a Tamil Hindu "mother goddess", embodying the universal principle of female energy (*cakti*). The fangs and crimson colour of this statue suggest the ferocity and "heat" of the goddess, while the children in her arms show her capacity to act as a nurturant and protective mother. From Rameswaram, Tamilnadu.

achieve puberty and sexual maturity through the same process that causes girls to begin to menstruate, but their maturation is considered to be more gradual. The cultural and emotional recognition of adult manhood occurs much later than adult womanhood, often as late as age 25 or 30. For one thing, males have less blood to spare, and there is great concern that male blood be conserved and utilized for later strength. The occurrance of seminal emissions among boys in adolescence is, like the start of menstruation for girls, an indication that the body has finally begun to produce excess blood. This follows the widespread South Asian belief that semen is a refined form, or as my informants put it, an "ambrosia" (*amirtam*) or a "distillation" (*vatippu*) of the blood, in accordance with a traditional ratio of volumes, usually 40 or 60 drops of blood producing one drop of semen. There seems to be no specific organ of seminal production except, perhaps, the brain itself, which is also the place where semen is stored and conserved.

The loss of semen through sex, masturbation, or nocturnal emission drains the body of valuable blood, while the retention of semen, particularly during adolescence and young manhood, promotes a man's physical, and ultimately his spiritual, development. The body of an ascetic young bachelor (*piramacāri*) should glow with good health. This agrees with fundamental South Asian yogic theory and was widely accepted by the young unmarried men I met during fieldwork. There is, in fact, an ominous proverb: *vintu vittān, nontu cettān,* "He spilled his semen; he was wounded and he died." The intensity of sexual desire is proportional to the rate of excess blood production and the amount of semen which has accumulated in the cranial reservoir, so in theory, a young man's desire entails its own incentive for asceticism (but see Carstairs, 1957, for the anxieties this may produce). Throughout the Tamil cultural area, the virtuous form of female control, which complements male sexual control, is "chastity" (*karpu*), implying supreme modesty and sexual fidelity. Hart (1973) has shown that the mystical power of female chastity (concentrated particularly in the breasts) has been a theme in Tamil literature since the first centuries A.D., while O'Flaherty (1969) has traced the intimate connection between ascetic and erotic ideals in Saivite mythology.

Through Puberty to Adulthood

For a girl, the passage into fertile, marriageable womanhood is, in principle, a cause for satisfaction and an opportunity to augur her future marriage and fertility. This passage also marks the beginning of the most stringent safeguards for her chastity and for the reputation of the whole family, since virginity is considered essential in a bride. There is ethnographic evidence which indicates that traditionally, despite some differences in the scale and content of the rituals, both Tamils and Moors celebrated female puberty in a broadly similar fashion, but today the two communities have quite different public reactions to the onset of menstruation. The Tamils extend their personal satisfaction into a conspicuous ritual celebration to which are invited neighbours, kinspeople, visiting anthropologists, indeed anyone within range of the blaring loudspeaker. The Moors, on the other hand, seem nowadays to be more concerned with the liabilities and proprieties of having a nubile unmarried daughter in the household, and so they avoid any public ritual which might draw attention to her changed status, particularly if they wish to keep her enrolled in a government school.

Tamil Rites of First Menstruation

A number of Tamil expressions for the ritual of first menstruation incorporate the word *kaliyāṇam,* which is also the most common term for wedding. A *kaliyāṇam* is actually any joyful, auspicious celebration, of which the epitome is a wedding. The auspiciousness of a daughter's entrance into womanhood, and the immediate connotations of marriageability which it suggests, account not only for the use of the expression *kaliyāṇam* but also for some of the explicit similarities between the puberty ritual and the wedding ritual. A formal observance of the rituals of first menstruation among the Tamils is often called a *rutukkaliyāṇam* (Tamil *irutu,* menstrual discharge), a *camarttiyakkaliyāṇam* (Tamil *camartti,* to fill or to complete), or simply a *periyappiḷḷaikkaliyāṇam,* "big girl *kaliyāṇam"*. People may say of a girl who has commenced to menstruate that she has "gotten big" (i.e. has matured), that she has "become knowledgeable", or that she has "flowered". A few brash young men were even heard to remark that such a girl was "fully cooked".[5]

Menstruation, along with birth and death, is considered to give rise to a temporary state of ritual pollution. A general word for such pollution among the Tamil Hindus is *tuṭakku,* and the roughly equivalent Moorish expression would be *muḻukku* (from *muḻuka,* to bathe completely). The pollution arising from the very first menstruation is considered to be especially severe, so one aim of the female puberty rituals is to contain and to remove this extraordinary contamination. A second aim of the rituals is to protect the newly matured girl from various malevolent forces, including voracious spirits and the evil eye, which pose extra hazards to the girl at this vulnerable transition-point in her life. A third goal served by the puberty rituals is to launch the girl into womanhood with the greatest degree of auspiciousness, celebration and good fortune, in the hope that these benign influences will carry over into later life. A fourth, but unstated, goal of these rituals is to advertize the marriageability of the nubile daughter, to activate promising kinship ties to marriageable cross-cousins and to demonstrate the wealth and standing of her family through conspicuous expenditure and generous hospitality for the invited guests. The Tamil Hindu ritual of first menstruation follows a basic sequence: (1) first indication, (2) first ritual bath, (3) seclusion period with special diet and protective measures, (4) second ritual bath and (5) domestic celebration.[6]

Reading the First Signs. The exact time of the onset of first menstruation is carefully noted, for it forms the basis of a necessary astrological computation to determine the auspicious time for the rituals which will conclude the period of seclusion and pollution. In some localities, astrological calculations also supply auspicious times for other parts of the ritual sequence. In every case, the astrologer will be expected to cast a horoscope for the puberty girl; this does not supplant the horoscope which is cast for every child at birth, but it does provide a "revised forecast" of the girl's marriage prospects, some vague clues as to the provenance and qualities of the likely groom and a projection of the number and sex of her offspring. It is considered inauspicious and unlucky for the girl to notice the first menstrual stains herself or for them to be noticed by a widow, an unmarried woman, or a man; it is best if they are first noticed by the girl's mother or by some other married woman with living children. There is a proverb: *tān kantāl kurram, tāy kantāl nallam,* "If you see it yourself it is a flaw, but if your mother sees it, it is a good thing".

A Quick Bath. The first ritual bath (*tannīr vārkiratu,* "pouring of water") generally takes place the very same day that the menstrual flow is detected: if formally commences the purification and ritual transformation of the girl. In rural Kokkatticcolai this is embellished with astrological computations and is announced with firecrackers in the streets, but in most parts of Batticaloa, the first bath is a hastily and quietly conducted affair with close kin and neighbours on hand to render assistance. The regular household Washerman of the Vannār caste is instructed to bring the necessary clean cloths and saris and to take away as a gift the polluted clothes worn by the girl when she began to menstruate. As a professional remover of pollution, the Washerman is an indispensible ritual specialist in puberty rites, and he stands to be generously remunerated with gifts of clothing, food and liquor.

A cloth is held up to shield the girl from onlookers while a group of *cumaṅkali*-s (auspicious, married women with living husbands and children) bring brass pots of water, mixed sometimes with turmeric and *aruku* grass, which one of the women then pours over the girl's head. There will be five or seven women, each with a pot, but there is no precise rule as to who they should be. Generally women such as the girl's mother's sister, her mother's brother's wife, or various "grannies" will serve in this role, but non-kinswomen are sometimes called; women of the girl's own household share her pollution and will not normally do this. There may be some variation between castes as to the degree of kin-role specification involved in this ritual. An untouchable Paraiyar Drummer with whom I spoke said that the bathing of the girl should be done specifically by her female cross-cousins, and Moorish sources said the same thing (see the section on "Moorish Rites in Comparison"). The bathing takes place on a plank and cloth laid on the ground not far from a doorway into the house, and men should avert their eyes. The girl deftly removes her soaked sarong, exchanges it for clean clothing brought by the Washerman, and is ushered into the house to begin her period of seclusion.

This first bath at least marks the beginning of her transition to womanhood and, as with other such beginnings (e.g. beginning of a new year), it is thought to augur well for the forthcoming enterprise if the first things the girl sees are beautiful, sacred and auspicious. Therefore, the girl will be asked to keep her eyes closed or downcast until she enters her seclusion room where she deliberately views a number of auspicious items which have been set out for her. This procedure is referred to as *kaṇ muḻikkiṟatu*, "opening the eyes" and glimpsing something lucky, such as a pot of water decorated with mango leaves and a coconut (*niṟai kuṭam*), a fresh coconut flower (spadix), or a gleaming oil lamp. Sometimes the first ritual bath mirrors in considerable detail the more fastidious conduct of the second ritual bath; both performances are felt to be essentially the same in terms of aim and content, but the second, being the culminating event, is typically more elaborated.

Pollution and Diet: Dangers of Hotness.   There is some degree of variation in the length of the seclusion period. In some localities the final bath takes place on or around the 31st day, which coincides with the standard Hindu pollution period for childbirth and death in the Batticaloa region. Other households are known to conduct the final bathing on the 7th, 9th, or 11th day in accordance with the astrologer's advice, which coincides more closely with the observance of ordinary menstrual pollution. In typical three-room houses facing east, the puberty girl occupies the northernmost room; in houses facing south, the easternmost room. This room is colloquially called the *cāyppūtu* ("sloping or leaning room", possibly referring to roof design or construction) or the *mañcūtu* ("bedroom"), and it is where childbirth also takes place traditionally. In the more isolated rural areas of Batticaloa, it is still the custom for members of the household to twist a length of paddystalk rope (*puri*) and fasten it across the yard to delineate the area of pollution at the northern or eastern end of the house. In addition, the Vaṇṇār Washerman ties a piece of white cloth to the roof of the house which serves as a visible warning to prospective callers. The girl is confined in her room with the shutters closed, but she has the constant company of the women and girls of her household and frequent visits by her girlfriends and female cousins. She must not be left alone, and she must take constant precautions against lurking spirits and sources of the evil eye. Spirits (*pēy, picācu*) are attracted by blood, particularly the "virgin blood" (*kaṇṇirattam*) of the puberty girl. A general-purpose prophylactic against spirits is iron, so the girl will carry an iron object, such as an arecanut cutter (*pākkuvetti*), on her person at all times, especially when she goes to the spirit-infested rear of the compound to urinate or defecate, or when she attends to ordinary bathing during the period of seclusion. The most common remedies for the evil eye are the drinking of water charmed with magical formulae and the display of marks and objects which catch the eye and serve as "lightning rods" for the evil eye. The evil eye (*kaṇṇūru, kaṇ patukiratu, tirushṭi*) can be transmitted unwittingly by anyone whose admiration or envy is aroused at a pleasant sight. This poses a dilemma for the puberty girl's family, whose desire to place the girl "on display" must be counterbalanced by attention to rituals which detract or remove the evil eye.

Diet for the girl during her seclusion period, and possibly for some time afterwards, is strictly controlled. Many of these foods are "cooling" in terms of their humoural value, and the cultural implication is that the girl is "hot". Blood is "hot", and the newly menstruating girl naturally picks up the heat of her overflowing blood, so one aim of the diet is to cool her body. There is also a desire to soothe her bleeding and to assist her "wound" to heal. For this, foods with *kiranti* (eruptive) quality are especially forbidden.[7] The ubiquitous tonic for the puberty girl is raw egg followed by an eggshell full of margosa oil administered right after the ritual baths, as well as intermittently during the seclusion period. All the products of the margosa tree (*Azadirachta indica*; Tamil *vēppamaram*) are cooling, but extremely bitter, so the oil (*vēppeṇṇey*) is commonly poured down the throat over a betel leaf after the egg has been swallowed. I was never given a complete theory of eggs, but they are considered to be very nutritious, probably a concentrated and re-fined form of blood akin to most reproductive fluids, and some people felt they had less gross humoural "heat" than meat. The consumption of raw eggs is always considered more nutritious than that of cooked eggs, and there is probably also an analogical assumption that, by eating raw eggs, the puberty girl will enhance her own fertility. No form of meat or fish is allowed during seclusion.

The particular form of carbohydrate favoured during the seclusion period is *pittu*, a compressed and steamed mixture of rice flour and grated coconut, to which is sometimes added a bit of black gram flour (*uluntu*). This steaming, crumbly *pittu* is a reasonably common form of breakfast food under any circumstances, but in the case of the puberty girl, it is mixed with sesame oil (*nallenney*) or margosa oil and wrapped up as a hot pack (*ottanam*) which is applied all around the girl's waist. She usually eats at least a bit of these hot packs afterwards, and every-one agrees that this treatment, together with the margosa oil, will lessen the girl's menstrual aches and cramps now and in the future. Although these packs are calorically hot, they are humourally "cool", and their purpose is to reduce the dangerous heat concentrated in her waist and loins.

Margosa, sesame and black gram are all "cooling" substances which are used in puberty seclusion. Except for eggs, the diet is completely vegetarian, with special favour shown towards relatively unspiced cur-ries made with tender (cool) vegetable sprouts (*piñcu*, e.g. green bean, eggplant, drumstick) and sesame oil instead of coconut milk. In fact, no milk or yoghurt of any kind is permitted, although some forms are admittedly very "cooling". The justification is vague, citing a tendency for milk to inhibit the healing of wounds or to cause diarrhoea. A number of highly eruptive (*kiranti*) foods, such as pineapple and cashew-fruit, were ruled out because they would clearly aggravate the "wound", and some kinds of tubers were also mentioned for their dangerous "windiness" (*vāyvu*). Whole kernels are considered the most nutritious form of rice, but foods cooked with rice flour are thought to be easier to digest, so the puberty girl receives lots of rice flour sweets, rice flour puddings and rice flour cakes. Chillies and other spices which are normally considered essential to the flavouring of curries are eliminated from the diet, too, because they are "heating". Salt is reduced or eliminated, but the only parallel I could find was with the elimination of salt from food offerings to the gods, where salt has associations with the mundane, the earthly. It may connote here simply a heightened sense of ritual occasion. Jaggary is favoured over refined sugar, apparently reflecting the fact that jaggary is cooling, while refined sugar is a modern product with no humoural valence in the traditional system. Turmeric in the form of paste is applied regularly to the girl's face and limbs; it is a very cooling substance felt to have value as a cosmetic (the yellow shade it imparts is seen as "whiteness") and as a medicine which counteracts pimples and blemishes. Its cooling and anti-eruptive qualities are also made use of in Hindu firewalking ceremonies, where the bodies of the devotees are smeared from head to toe with tumeric paste, and it is a very common purifying substance in Hindu ritual generally (Beck, 1969, p. 559).

Kaliyāṇam: Final Bath and Celebration. The day and exact time of the final ritual bath are authorized by the astrologer, and it is the events which transpire on this occasion which justify the term "wedding" (*kaliyāṇam*). The house is purified by sprinkling tumeric water and, traditionally, smearing a fresh coat of cow dung on the floor. The house is then decorated with the hereditary marks of honour (*varicai*) associated with different castes and matriclans, and in front of the house a *pantal* (temporary framework of wood and cloth) has been erected to shelter the guests. These are duties traditionally performed by the Washerman, but I have also seen the job done by members of the household, and in one case entirely by women, who were having a very gay time of it. This is an event in which women enact the major roles and men are either supporting players (e.g. the Vaṇṇār Washerman) or detached onlookers and guests. At the auspicious moment, the girl is led out of the house to the spot where the basic sequence of the first ritual bath is repeated, but with generally greater attention to detail. This time the auspicious women who carry the pots of water may make a point of filling the pots silently and reverently, they often bring the pots in a mini-procession under a cloth canopy (*mērkaṭṭi*), and they may each wear a white cloth on their head, supplied by the Washerman. These or similar cloths will be used to cover the mouths of the full water pots prior to the bath. One or more of the pots will contain *mañcanīr* (tumeric water with *aruku* grass) and possibly a bit of sea water (also purifying). Sometimes a herbal infusion-pack (*arappu*), prescribed by the astrologer to counteract unfavourable planetary influences (*kirakatōsham*), will be placed on the girl's head while the water is poured. The custom is no longer always observed, but traditionally in the Akkaraipattu area a full measure (*marakkāl*) of paddy and a quarter measure (*niṟainaḷi*) of rice should be placed beside the bathing spot to be taken away by the Washerman along with the wet bathing garment.[8]

In the Kokkatticcolai area the custom is to circle five or seven boxes containing *piṭṭu* (steamed rice flour and coconut) and *kaḷi* (rice flour pudding) around the girl's head immediately upon completion of her bath. Ritually, these boxes of food transfer lingering pollution and evil eye from the puberty girl to the Washerman, but they also constitute one of the major payments for the Washerman's services. For this reason, the ritual of the final day is referred to in this area as the *piṭṭu kaḷi celavu*, "*piṭṭu* and *kaḷi* expenditure".

At this point, if not earlier, the puberty girl is joined by a much younger girl, usually one of her cross-cousins, who has been designated her "companion girl" (*tōḻippeṇ*) and whose duty it is to accompany the girl everywhere as a sort of walking decoy for the evil eye. Once the girl has hastily donned some clean, dry clothing, she is ready to celebrate her new status by dressing as a mature woman in an elegant sari and borrowed jewelry for the first time. She also must be presented with the *ālātti*, a series of decorated tapers which are lit and circled around her body to detract and remove the evil eye. And she must make her ceremonial first entrance into the house as a mature woman and have another "auspicious first glimpse" of the items set out for this purpose. In one instance, I saw that she was given yet another dose of margosa oil and raw egg, plus sesame oil, a bit of turmeric paste and, finally, betel leaf and arecanut to chew to remove the awful taste from her mouth. The sequence of these final events, however, can vary a good deal. I have seen the *ālātti* tapers waved around the girl while she remained standing on the bathing plank, and I have seen them waved after she has been completely dressed in her formal sari and jewelry. In general, the *ālātti* immediately precedes what is deemed to be the ceremonial first entrance of the new woman into the house through the front door, in spite of the fact that she may have dodged into the rear of the house to get dressed. There will be five or seven or nine *ālātti*-s, usually a sequence of colourfully decorated designs in dough, each with a decreasing number of wicks imbedded. A suitable senior woman, perhaps one who helped with the bathing, waves each burning *ālātti* in front of and around the girl, then sets it aside for the Washerman to take away. There is enormous variety in the types of *ālātti*-s fashioned by women of different households, but they are all presented in an order of diminishing brilliance, with the aim of drawing the evil eye away from the girl and then extinguishing it. The girl sometimes then tosses two betel leaves backwards over her shoulder to further jettison the evil eye and walks immediately into the house on a carpet of pure cloths laid down by the Washerman. Once she is inside the house, has completed her auspicious glimpse, and has eaten her prescribed foods, she is put on display in all her finery. A temporary decorated seat is provided for the girl and her *tōḻippeṇ*, and together they receive the gifts and felicitations of the guests who have come to the celebration. Nowadays even poor households will seek to hire a loudspeaker to advertize the happy event with well-worn cinema music, and in some places drummers and shawm-players of the Naṭṭuvar Musician caste are booked for the occasion. A full meal of rice and curry is prepared for the guests, and the household basks in satisfaction at the removal of the girl's pollution and her emergence as a woman. Throughout the seclusion period, and during the celebration of the final bath, it is expected that the girl's female cross-cousins (her mother's brother's daughters, father's sister's daughters, and classificatory extensions) will indulge in some lighthearted "turmeric-play" (*mañcaḷ vilaiyāṭṭu*) amongst themselves when they visit the house, and this may be duplicated amongst cross-cousins in the parental generation, too. Although I never witnessed much of this, it was at least widely joked about, and it reflects the heightened awareness of possible marriage connections with the girl's potential sisters-in-law. A modern touch which is sometimes added to the whole affair in recent years is the distribution of formal printed invitations to attend the puberty ceremony. In such instances, the language of the invitation is suitably elevated, and the ceremony itself might be billed, for example, as a "sacred ameliorative water-anointment" (*tiru cānti nīrāṭṭam*).

There are a number of explicit parallels between the puberty rituals and the Tamil Hindu wedding rites which any one will happily point out. The house is decorated in the same manner as for a wedding and is loosely called a "wedding house" (*kaliyāṇa vīṭu*). The attire of the newly purified puberty girl is often as lavish as a bride's, and the sari is often the appropriate colour (red or pink). The waving of the *ālātti* and the tossing of betel leaves occurs in all weddings just prior to the ceremonial entrance of the bride and groom into the house. In fact, the house at which both rituals take place is often the same, since marriage is matri-uxorilocal. Once inside, the puberty girl sits upon a specially decorated seat called, figuratively, a "wedding chamber" (*maṇavarai*), just as the bride and groom do after their nuptials. The puberty girl has her cross-cousin "companion girl" or "bridesmaid" (*tōḷippeṇ*) who safeguards her, and a bridegroom has his male cross-cousin "groom's companion" (*māppiḷḷai tōḷan*) who accompanies him in procession to the bride's house for the wedding. In the most elaborate puberty ceremony I ever witnessed, the sari to be worn by the girl after her final bath was brought in procession with musical accompaniment from her father's sister's house, and the sari was carried in a *kūṟaippeṭṭi* (bridal sari box) along with boxes of sweets just as it would have been carried by the groom's party to the bride's house for a wedding. At the gateway to the girl's household compound, a customary "meeting"

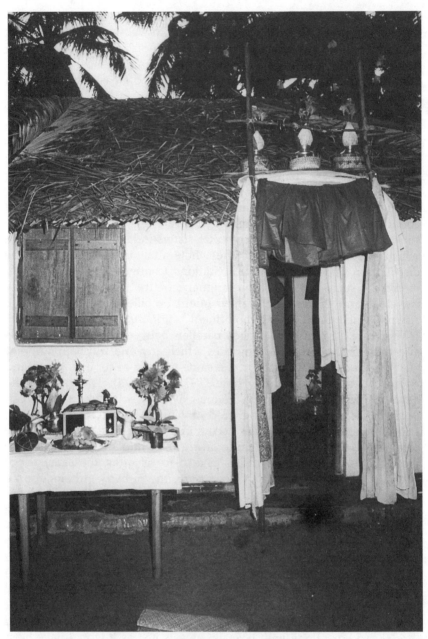

Fig. 3.   A house decorated for the final stage of a Tamil Hindu girl's ritual of first menstruation in eastern Sri Lanka. Cloths and brass pots over the doorway indicate her family's caste and clan status as well as underscoring the symbolism of re-entry into the house as a mature woman. Items on the table, including a new transistor radio, are a combination of the auspicious and the decorative.

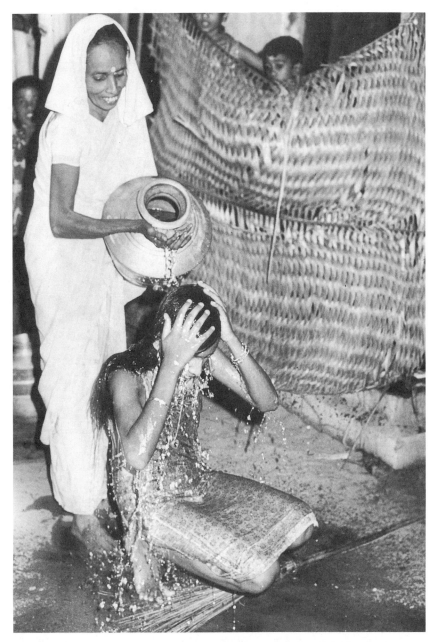

Fig. 4. An auspicious married woman with living husband and children is chosen to pour the water during the girl's final ritual bath. Usually seven pots of water are drawn from the well, and the bathing takes place in a temporary enclosure beside the house. In some households the girl stands on a rake as extra protection against lurking spirits.

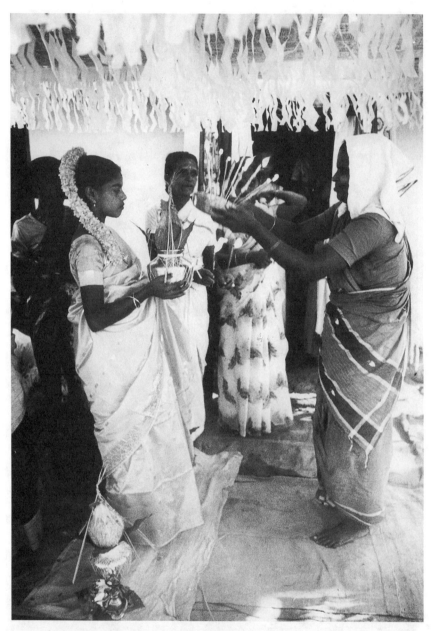

Fig. 5. After the final bath, the girl is dressed for the first time in full mature women's attire. Insofar as possible, she is made to look like a bride, with a pink or red bridal sari and heavy gold jewelry. Here, the adorned girl holds an auspicious *kumpam* pot, while the older women wave the *ālātti* (a sequence of lighted tapers) to honour her and to draw away the evil eye, as would also be done at a wedding.

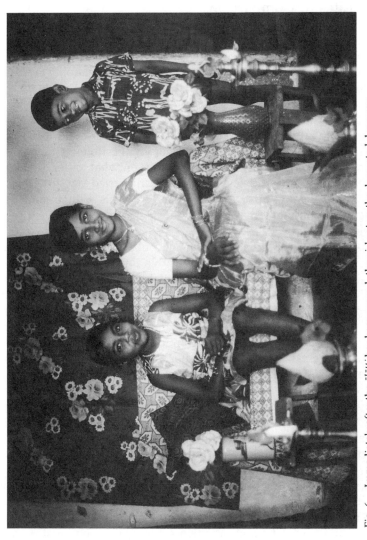

Fig. 6. Immediately after the *ālāti* has been waved, the girl enters the decorated doorway of the house a purified and fertile woman: she is accompanied during the rituals by her "companion girl", a young female cross-cousin who insures that she is never alone and who serves to detract the evil eye from the puberty girl herself. Inside the house they sit on a decorated throne and receive gifts and greetings from relatives and well-wishers, including potential affines.

ritual (*cantippu*) to hand over the sari was staged between two women, one representing the group bringing the sari and the other representing the girl's household, just as occurs at a wedding celebration.

Moorish Rites in Comparison

The prospects of finding a quick and suitably prestigious match for one's nubile daughters are increasingly dim these days for both the Tamils and the Moors, and this is reflected in the rising national average age of women at marriage. But while the Tamils seem to feel that a daughter's puberty is both an auspicious rite of passage and an opportunity for her to "come out" publicly as a marriageable woman, the Moors seem to treat it, publicly at least, as an embarrassment. Moorish people with whom I spoke, who were generally wealthier farmers and professionals, voiced anxiety at the thought of what other families would say of them, having several mature unmarried daughters still sitting at home. I knew just as many Hindu Tamils with unmarried daughters, but while they may have felt despair, they did not express such a feeling of shame.

There is no public observance of female puberty rituals among the Moors in the major coastal settlements at this time as far as I am able to determine, but older people clearly remembered the ceremonies during their lifetime. Historical data is difficult to obtain, but I suspect that Moorish modesty about female puberty has grown in recent years in response to the spread of greater pan-Islamic consciousness. There is a feeling, particularly among the more middle-class Moorish families, that Islamic respectability requires greater attention to the seclusion of women, and this naturally makes the Tamil female puberty ceremony seem, in contrast, like an immodest spectacle. In the wake of intermittent Hindu/Muslim communal riots in parts of the Batticaloa region in recent years, the Moors have also deliberately banned some traditional customs which seemed to link them too closely with "Hindu" cultural practices. Female puberty ceremonies may have been influenced by this tension. Having adopted a general strategy of modesty and seclusion towards their mature daughters, the Moors can only be tempted to intensify this trend in face of an unfavourable marriage market. There is very little scope for the employment of Moorish women outside the home except among the poorest families, who must permit their women to work in weeding brigades in the paddy fields or in handloom workshops. A daughter's first menstruation is now a source of chagrin to Moorish parents who would prefer to keep her in school or who would prefer that she could travel more freely. One solution is simply to keep quiet about menarche and hope that the gossip can be minimized.

The traditional Moorish rituals of first menstruation, as described by various people, are simpler than those for the Tamils, but they are basically similar in terms of the overall sequence, the supernatural safeguards and the special diet given to the girl. On the other hand, the kinship and affinal implications of the event are given more explicit emphasis. Both the first and the second bath are administered by the girl's female cross-cousins but are not particularly ritualized. The Moorish girl's terminological (and potentially real) mothers-in-law (*māmī*), in other words her mother's brother's wife, father's sister and their classificatory equivalents, are described specifically as crucial figures in the Moorish puberty observances, while the Tamils, both in theory and in practice, are less explicit about this and seem a bit more flexible about kin-role participation. In the Moorish puberty sequence, the mother's brother's wife and the father's sister are expected to bring much of the food and raw material consumed during the girl's seclusion period. Various people described the Moorish puberty observance as an occasion when promising marriage connections with specific cross-cousins were deliberately cultivated by the girl's family, who would send special boxes of *piṭṭu* and sweets (*ceppu*) to these households after the completion of the final bath. The idea of "tumeric-play" between female cross-cousins at the puberty house was also vividly recalled. Occasionally even a male cross-cousin was doused with the yellow pigment, and often the mischief spread to senior generations, with various grannies stalking each other at a slower pace.

From a ritual point of view, the Moorish observance of first menstruation represents a trimmed-down version of what the Tamils do, except for a few unique embellishments. The sequence of first indication, first bath, seclusion and final bath is similar, and the dietary rules are just the same. Notice of a girl's initial menstruation by a widow is considered quite harmful. The only clearly Islamic element in the entire event is the recitation of the *kālimā* ("There is no God but Allah, and Mohammed is His Prophet") by the puberty girl when she first becomes aware of her menstruation. This is the procedure to be followed at all subsequent menstruations, and it marks the beginning of the period of pollution which bars a menstruating woman from fasting, from reciting her daily prayers, or from touching the Holy Koran. The timing of the second bath, which ends the period of pollution for a Moorish puberty girl, is ascertained by the Muslim priest (Lebbe, *ilavvai*) using standard divination techniques involving the counting of betel leaves and arecanuts or using a numerological computation based upon the girl's mother's name. The usual period of seclusion is said to be seven or nine days, during which the girl is never left alone and never allowed to venture outside the house without an object of iron, or a broomstick, to ward off spirits. She is given the same doses of raw egg, margosa oil and other cooling substances as a Tamil girl is given, and she also eats *piṭṭu* and is given hot packs of *piṭṭu* around her waist. The girl's final bath is performed by her cross-cousins while she sits on a low stool covered with white cloth, betel leaves and arecanut. The betel and arecanut are afterwards tossed on to the roof of the house. After the bath, the Moorish girl may be given an auspicious first glimpse of a mound of tumeric paste decorated with lighted wicks or a pot of water surmounted by a coconut flower. The *ālātti* used by the Moors at puberties and weddings is a permanent object of wood, tinsel and coloured paper resembling a minature Christmas tree. One or more *ālātti*-s are waved about the puberty girl by her female cross-cousins and are then returned to their owners for re-use.

Moorish families do not seem to have followed the Tamil custom of exhibiting the newly matured puberty girl in elaborate clothing on a special decorated "marriage chamber" seat, but they definitely required the girl to take three sips of *pāl palam*, a mixture of mashed banana, coconut milk and sugar which is administered in similar fashion to both Tamil and Moorish brides and grooms after the wedding necklace (*tāli*) has been tied.[9] Some Moors also testified that firecrackers and *kuravai* (women's shrill joyous warbling) would announce to the neighbourhood the completion of the girl's final purification and attainment of maturity, just as they would customarily announce the arrival of the groom's party at the bride's gate.

Ordinary Menstruation

Sometimes the puberty girl continues to receive doses of raw egg and margosa oil during several subsequent menstrual periods, in order to ensure that her menstrual cramps will not be severe in later life. On these occasions she may also be rubbed with turmeric paste to promote smooth skin and light complexion. As menstruation becomes a routine part of a woman's life, however, the ritual observances and the behavioural restrictions are reduced. The first basic restriction which is observed by most families today is that a menstruating wife or daughter must sleep apart from her ordinary bedroom or sleeping place, and keep away from her husband if she is married. In practice this means sleeping in an outer room or in a separate structure, and using separate sleeping mats or burlap sacks for temporary bedding. Some older people mentioned special menstrual seclusion huts in the rear of the household compound, but there is no evidence of this practice today, and it is difficult to know how widespread it once was. Nowadays, a menstruating woman might simply move her sleeping place to an outer room or to an already existing shed. The arrangements involve an *ad hoc* compromise between the desire to separate the polluted woman and the concern that she be sheltered from prowling spirits who would be attracted to blood. The second basic restriction which is observed today is the rule that a menstruating woman must not draw water from a well; if she does it is said that the well water will become infested with worms (*pulu*). Many people will also state that the woman should not cook, but there seems to be tacit agreement that this is a more flexible rule. A menstruating woman should also avoid sitting on chairs or benches, but since women generally tend to stand or squat, this usually poses no extra inconvenience.

No special dietary rules are invoked during ordinary menstruation; the main concern is with the woman's state of temporary menstrual pollution, which typically lasts a week. In general terms, this is another instance of the same ritual pollution which arises at childbirth and at death and which is commonly called *tuṭakku*. One may allude or refer to the menstrual condition by terms such as *tīṭṭu* (this is rare, but refers specifically to menstrual pollution), *māta viṭāy* ("monthly weariness"), *tuvālai* (menstrual discharge), *talai muḻukkiṟatu* ("dousing the head" i.e. taking the required full bath), *vīṭṭukku tūram* ("away from the house", i.e. menstrual isolation), or simply *ākātu* ("not possible, not allowed", i.e. to act normally). For Moors, the general pollution category of *muḻukku* also covers menstrual impurity, and generally the same types of domestic restrictions on menstrual women are noted in Moorish households, although it was more difficult for me to obtain precise information. Needless to say, both Tamil and Moorish women are required to suspend formal religious activities, such as attending temple pūjas or reciting Muslim prayers, until after menstrual pollution is removed. Unless special isolation precautions are taken, menstrual pollution will also negate the efficacy of beneficial charms or mantras being recited in the house. The first three days of a woman's menstrual period are considered to be the most severely polluting, but in any case a full "head bath" is required by both the Hindus and the Muslims in order to return the woman to a normal state. The standard procedure for Muslim ablutions prior to daily prayers, or after sexual intercourse, involves a set of invocations for each step in the washing sequence. I was told that Moorish women should also perform these ablutions as part of their final menstrual bath, but I do not know whether this is typically done. The ritual emphasis during ordinary menstruation is on pollution, rather than bodily heat, but the underlying connection between these two in South Asian thought has already been well established (Beck, 1969; Babb, 1975).

Male Rites of Passage

The belief that boys mature more slowly than girls is reflected in relatively late observance of the traditional Tamil male rite of passage into adulthood, somewhere between the ages of 16 and 22. This ritual is no longer performed, and only older people could offer a description of it. The common name for the ritual was *kātukkuttukirakkaliyāṇam* ("ear-piercing *kaliyāṇam*") or *kaṭukkaṇpoṭukirakkaliyāṇam* ("ear-stud placing *kaliyāṇam*"). The timing of the ceremony seems to have been determined by convenience, although astrological factors were probably also taken into account. Formerly a young man's beard would never have been shaved until the day of this ceremony, when the family Barber would come to the house for this purpose. Then the man would bathe, washing his head and face with young coconut water (*iḷanīr*) and turmeric water, which are both "cooling" fluids, and his hair would be tied into the traditional male bun (*koṇṭai* or *kuṭumi*) for the first time. Next, the goldsmith would step forward to pierce the man's ears and insert the male gold ear-studs (*kaṭukkaṇ*), which signify male adulthood. Finally, the man would be dressed in a fine new white cloth (*vēṭṭi*), shawl (*cālvai*) and turban (*talaippā*) and be taken to the front of the house where *ālātti* wicks would be waved around him and, possibly, baskets of fried sweets (*palakāram*) and parched grain (*pori*) poured over his head. He would then be considered a *kaṭukkeṉṟavaṉ*, a grown man eligible to marry.[10]

I have come across no evidence that Moorish youths underwent such an explicit ritual of adult manhood, although the attitudes and expectations associated with a delayed entrance into adulthood are shared by both Moors and Tamils. Although Muslim circumcision would seem at first the obvious parallel ritual, in fact it is performed well before what is believed to be the age of sexual maturity (i.e. it is performed around the age of 9 or 10). Moorish sources indicate that, technically, circumcision should be done in infancy (as with the female incision, see the section on Final Purifications, Protections and Practices), but parents prefer to wait until later, when the boy is more likely to survive the operation. Nevertheless, Muslim circumcision (*cuṉṉattu*) conforms in many ways to the symbolic model of the wedding: the event is still called *cuṉṉattukkaliyāṇam*, and traditionally the boy was elaborately

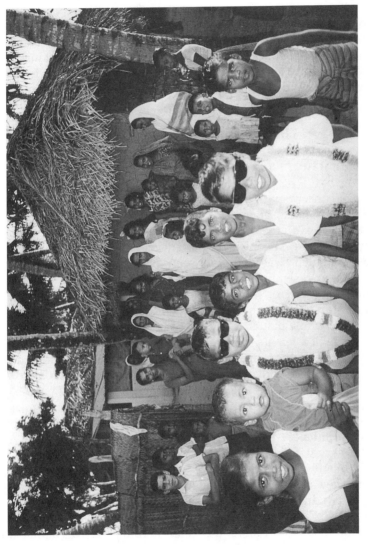

Fig. 7.   Among the Moors of eastern Sri Lanka, several boys may be circumcised in a single ceremony, commonly referred to as a "circumcision wedding". In this photo the two boys wearing garlands and sunglasses are enjoying the gifts and compliments of well-wishers before they undergo the operation.

decorated and taken in procession through the village before the operation was performed. An informal appellation for the boy is cuṉṉattu māppiḷḷai, "circumcision bridegroom" and, as with all weddings, wealthier families today distribute printed invitations.[11] There are also striking similarities between the regimen and diet of the convalescing circumcision boy and those of the secluded puberty girl: eggs, cooling oils, piṭṭu (also applied in hot packs), cooling leaf curries (cuntal), a ban on meat, fish and milk products, plus the usual precautions against lurking spirits. The period of seclusion and convalescence for the boy is concluded with a special bath initiated by the specialist circumciser himself.

The Reproductive Process

Conception: The Two Semens

Theories of conception in the Batticaloa region contend that a woman is fertilized when male semen (cukkilam, intiriyam, vintu, tātu, kāmappāl etc.) mixes in the uterus with female semen (curōṇitam, nātam, but frequently unnamed). People were often vague about the nature of female semen, but it was definitely seen as derived from blood and was assumed to resemble male semen. They said it came from the head, from the chest, or from the womb itself; some felt that it was less important in conception than male semen, and a few people were ignorant of the whole matter. Only four out of the sample of 35 denied any knowledge of a female substance involved in conception, and only one raised the metaphor of the male "seed" emplanted in the female "field" as recorded in Indian ethnography (Mayer, 1960, p. 203; Fruzzetti and Östör, 1976; Dube, 1978) and in the Laws of Manu (IX, 31–56). Typically, the paired expression cukkilacurōṇitam was widely recognized as representing the two essential substances in conception, and this accords with Sinhalese belief as well (Obeyesekere, 1976, p. 207). Although the sexual fluids are refined essences likened to "ambrosia" (amirtam) while they are stored in the body, in the aftermath of sexual intercourse they are treated as polluting. To remove the temporary pollution of Hindus who have had sexual relations during the night, a full "head-bath" is required the following morning before any clean tasks are undertaken; for Moors, the technical rule prescribes a full bath immediately afterwards, as well as between repeated acts of intercourse. Some Moorish people told me, however, that this was carrying things a bit too far.

Fertilization occurs with the mixing of the sexual fluids during that part of a woman's monthly cycle when her uterine "flower" (as it is commonly expressed) is in bloom and can provide an opening to admit them. This opening is generally believed to close two weeks after the end of the previous menstrual flow. The heat of sexual desire "melts" the semi-solid reservoir of semen in the brain, allowing it to flow downward, in some accounts via the spinal column and intermediate storage sacs in the naval or testes, to the penis.[12] This process illuminates one of the rarer terms for male semen: *kāmappāl*, "milk of lust". For fertilization to occur, both sexual partners must achieve orgasm. This is necessary because both sexual fluids must be ejaculated into the womb, where they mix to produce the beginnings of an embryo, variously described as a bubble (*kumili*), a lump (*katti*), or a sprout (*mulai*). One man offered a precise ethno-chemical explanation: male semen is salty (*uppu*) and female semen is sour (*puli*). Just as salt water mixed with sour tamarind water will produce a solid coagulum, so male and female semen will curdle to form the embryo (*karu*). Although this theory seemed eccentric at the time, I later found support for it in a Tamil classification of "male" alkaline substances (*āncarakku*) and "female" acidic substances (*pencarakku*), otherwise referred to as *uppuvintu* (male seminal salts) and *puliccurōnitam* (female seminal acids, i.e. "sour" *curōnitam*).[13] A few people, mostly curing specialists, added that the three Ayurvedic humours, and particularly the *pirāna vāyvu* (wind of life), would be present at conception. If a specific source of *uyir* (life, spirit) could be specified, it was invariably the *pirāna vāyvu*, which pervades the womb from the surrounding universe and has no connection with either parent.[14]

I was also informed of a haphazard assortment of ancillary factors which were conducive to successful impregnation, ranging from unity of mind, to simultaneous orgasm, to hydraulically forceful ejaculation. The main point, however, is that conception is seen by most people fundamentally bilateral, involving substances from both parents. Few specific characteristics of the child are determined at the point of conception itself, except for the sex of the child. I heard five different theories of how the sex of the child is determined at conception, depending on (1) whether intercourse takes place on even (male) versus odd (female) days following the end of menstrual pollution, (2) whether the parents are breathing through the right (male) versus left (female) nostril at the moment of fertilization, (3) whether the mother sleeps on her right (male) or left (female) side after intercourse, (4) whether the first sexual fluid to enter the womb is from the father or from the mother, (5) whether a relatively greater amount of male or female semen is deposited in the womb. Some curing practitioners claimed to be able to utilize *kaippiṭi vaittiyam* ("hand-holding medicine", sphygmology) in order to ascertain the sex of the foetus by comparing the strength of the pulse in the pregnant woman's right (male) versus left (female) wrist. Twins or multiple births are not clearly explained in local theory, although repeated intercourse the same night is one hypothesis offered. The birth of twins is not given much significance: it is an abnormality, so it may suggest some sort of flaw or blemish (*kuṟṟam*), but for the most part, it is just seen as an additional burden on the mother.

Gestation: Transfer of Blood

Within the womb, the child is said to be nourished by a direct blood transfusion from the mother via the opening (*tuvāram*) which all foe-tuses are said to have at the top of the head. As tangible proof, people cited the soft area of the newborn child's cranium, the fontanelle, which they said represented the recently closed channel by which maternal blood had reached the foetus.[15] Because the contribution of bodily sub-stance from the mother is seen as a massive and prolonged diversion of her own blood, and because the matrilineal and matrilocal social institutions of the Batticaloa region tend to foster a "matrilateral bias" in local thinking, many of my friends disagreed radically with the common South Asian belief, which is particularly associated with pa-trilineal ideology and institutions, that the child's blood is a perpetua-tion of the father's blood transmitted in the form of male semen. The conflict between the matrilineal traditions and beliefs of Batticaloa peo-ple and the patrilineal ideology which nowadays impinges from the larger South Asian cultural environment (and from patrilineal Jaffna and Tamilnadu in particular) was reflected in the pattern of responses to my question concerning the identity of the child's blood. Although the question, as I posed it, had scarcely occurred to many people, their opinions soon sharply and evenly divided three ways. Some, who had earlier stressed the potency of male semen in conception, said that semen was a concentrated form of the father's blood which the child consequently shared. Others vehemently objected to this view, saying that the tiny amount of father's semen was insignificant in comparison to the mother's massive transference of blood to the child during preg-nancy and lactation; the child's blood was definitely that of the mother, according to this second view. The third group more closely followed the local theory of conception, pointing out that both parents contribute elements of their bodily substance, so that the child's blood must be a bilateral composite of the mother's and the father's blood. Whatever their views on this question, all agreed that the subsequent gestation and development of the embryo after conception draw solely upon the bodily resources (blood) of the mother. Continued intercourse during the early part of pregnancy is allowed. However, it has no effect of nourishing or augmenting the embryo, and if continued for too long, it threatens the health of the foetus by generating excessive heat.[16] All in all, the fleeting quality of the paternal role in impregnation, as contrasted with the maternal burden of carrying and nourishing the child through pregnancy, is well recognized in the local proverb: *aiyāvukku aintu nimisham, ammāvukku pattu mātam*, "Five minutes for the father, ten months for the mother".

Menstruation ceases with pregnancy because the "excess blood" normally eliminated during the monthly period now goes to nourish the foetus. There is a belief that menstrual blood is extremely polluting, yet the uterine blood which flows to the child is beneficial. People were unsure on this point: one man said that bodily impurities were carried away by the flow of the menstrual blood, making it a bad or unclean fluid (*turnīr*) analogous to sweat, urine and faeces, whereas this excretory function ceased during pregnancy. Another person hastily reasoned that impure menstrual blood must be stored in a separate sac during pregnancy to be discharged with the afterbirth. Many, supporting ideas put forward by Mary Douglas, said that menstrual blood, like certain other bodily substances (saliva, semen, hair) only becomes polluting when it leaves the boundary of the body (Douglas, 1966). This latter interpretation provides the most satisfactory explanation, since it fits a wide range of South Asian bodily pollution beliefs, and also accords with indigenous thinking on the subject.

There are relatively few strict rules concerning the diet and behaviour of a woman during pregnancy. Naturally enough, it is felt that she should eat an especially nutritious diet so that her body can restore the blood which is continuously passing into the foetus. She should eat "normally" (*cātāranamāka*), I was told, taking into account the same sorts of humoural balances a non-pregnant woman would observe. When pressed further, some people cautioned against excessive amounts of "cooling, eruptive, or windy" foods, all of which might threaten the stability of the foetus according to local reasoning. However, no clearly defined antenatal diet appears to exist; most informants mentioned rice, vegetables, milk products, eggs, meat and fish as "foods which would cause fresh blood to seep forth" (*irattattai ūrutarkuriya cāppātu*). It is the custom to bring a newly pregnant woman a type of plump steamed tart with sweet filling called *kolukkattai* ("fat block"), occasionally even one which contains another smaller tart within it (*pillaikkolukkattai*, "child *k.*"). These are also commonly exchanged sweets at weddings, where their auspicious "plump" health and fertility symbolism is equally appropriate. The only strongly proscribed foods and substances fall into the category of abortifacients, all of which seem to possess excessive levels of *kiranti* (eruptive) quality. The most commonly mentioned food in this category is pineapple (*annācippaḻam*), but an intentional combination of other *kiranti* foods (e.g. prawns, *kiri* fish, *māci* dried fish, eggplant, papaya, guavas, *kuruttu* coconut sprout etc.) would also pose a danger to the foetus. In order to induce an abortion, it was said that a woman might surreptitiously consume several pineapples, or she might even take a bit of stinging jellyfish (*cori muṭṭai*, "itch eggs"), which is the most potent abortifacient of all. However, all my informants expressed the opinion that abortion was a deplorable practice, a heinous sin.

Pregnancy cravings (*icā*) are a recognized aspect of pregnancy, but they are much less culturally elaborated than among the Kandyan Sinhalese studied by Obeyesekere (1963). The commonly reported pregnancy cravings in Batticaloa are for sour foods (green mangos, tamarind, limes), bitter substances (*vipūti* sacred ash, burnt rice from the bottom of the pot) and sweet things (*palakāram* fried cakes, *muttāci* sweets). Most people find these cravings amusing and easy to satisfy, and there is no evidence that pregnancy cravings serve to channel resentment of female childbearing and male dominance (c.f. Obeyesekere's analysis of Sinhalese pregnancy cravings). Given the matrilineal and matrilocal social organization in Batticaloa, and the absence of the severe wife abuse Obeyesekere reports from Kandyan areas, such a result is not surprising. The ethnomedical explanation of pregnancy cravings is that they are generated when the nutritional demands of the foetus excessively tax the nutritional resources of the mother, and a general response (in addition to satisfying the cravings themselves) is to augment the mother's diet in all respects.

Most people seem to have no clear idea of exactly how the foetus develops in the uterus, but there are traditional medical songs which a number of Ayurvedic curing specialists recited in response to my questions on this topic. These verses are mainly descriptive, as opposed to diagnostic, in nature, and the singing usually a bit rusty, but all the songs attempt to specify characteristic stages of foetal development for each month of gestation.[17] None of the recitations I heard matched perfectly, but the general sequence starts with the embryonic lump (sprout, bubble etc.), which develops shoulders and a nape by the first or second month, head, torso, and limbs by the third or fourth month, bodily orifices by the fifth or sixth month, internal organs, blood vessels and nerves (*nāṭi*), joints and hair by the seventh or eighth month. By the ninth month, the child's body is complete: it then acquires the umbilical cord (*mākkoṭi, pokkaṇikkoṭi*) through which it receives actual food (chyme) from the mother's stomach, and the cranial blood orifice grows shut. At this point, it is time for the child to acquire consciousness (*aṟivu*) and to prepare for what lies ahead: in an upright foetal position (perceived as a gesture of worship) the baby prays to God and contemplates his karmic destiny in this rebirth. Then the *apāna vāyvu*, the special downward humoural wind, which guards the foetus and "drives" the processes of birth, menstruation and excretion, flips the foetus over so that it is head down and in position for labour to start. This humoural wind then expels the neonate into the world, although an insufficiency of the *apāna vāyvu* may result in a breech birth.

The Secrecy of Birth

Childbirth at home takes place in the northern or eastern room (*mañcūṭu*) of the traditional Tamil house. Moorish practice is similar, although Moorish houseplans are less uniform. Nowadays, however, it is becoming fairly common for childbirth to take place in local or regional government hospitals, and the traditional role of the midwife is gradually fading. Feeling about hospital births seems mixed: on the one hand, the maternity ward is unfamiliar, far from one's supportive kinswomen, and the hospital standard of care may have its shortcomings; on the other hand, hospital delivery lifts a messy, highly polluting and somewhat embarrassing event out of the household altogether, and the relative advantages of hospital medicine are increasingly accepted. A desire for privacy and isolation are major concerns: in fact, the specially built maternity hospital in an exposed location near the centre of Akkaraipattu town has been forced to close for lack of patients, while the relatively isolated (indeed, for most medical problems, quite inaccessible) government hospital several miles out of town draws a steady stream of maternity cases. Until fairly recently, childbirth at home was a common practice, and so I found that information about traditional customs was easy to elicit. I should state, however, that because hospital births are now common, and because the whole business of childbirth is an exclusively female domain, I never saw an actual childbirth nor witnessed the events immediately surrounding it.

The traditional midwife (*maruttuvicci*) is a woman from one of the lower service castes, most often from the Washerman (*Vaṇṇār*) or Barber (*Nāvitar*) castes, but in recent times there have also been government-trained midwives from other groups. Nevertheless, the midwife role clearly conforms with the domestic pollution-removing functions of the

Washerman and the Barber.[18] The other central figure is of course the woman's mother, assisted by other experienced kin and neighbourhood women. When the waters break, all men of the household leave the house and remain some distance away until the child is born. Childbirth is deemed an appalling sight which no man should witness, while the possibility of severe ritual pollution acts as a further deterrent. The techniques of the actual delivery are not secret, but they are so deeply shrouded in female modesty that I was unable to learn much about them, except that the woman often labours in a seated position against a sack of paddy.

The childbirth house is completely shuttered and closed during the actual delivery and during much of the postnatal pollution period. As in the period of seclusion during first menstruation, this is done in order to protect the mother and baby from marauding spirits, ghosts and demons which are attracted to all the blood and contamination. All of the same anti-demonic safeguards are prescribed, especially having the woman carry an iron object on her person at all times. There is also an effort to avoid drawing the attention of spirits and malevolent forces to the child; this means that notification of the birth should be done indirectly. Instead of shouting the sex of the child, a message is sent to the father requesting him to come immediately to the house and to toss a paddy pestle (ulakkai) over the top of the house if it is a boy, or a rake (īkkil kaṭṭi) if it is a girl. I was also told that tossing these symbolic objects would promote the child's later manly or womanly qualities. No external notification of any kind is given until after the umbilical cord has been cut and tied; if the sex of the child is acknowledged before this is done, both mother and child are placed in grave danger. Later, neighbours, kinsmen and friends are indirectly notified of the birth by the presentation of rock candy (karkaṇṭu) if it is a boy, jaggary (cakkarai) if it is a girl.

The birth horoscope of each child must eventually be calculated, so it is essential that the exact time of the birth (technically the moment when the head can first be seen) is recorded.[19] For the Hindus, the birth horoscope is used in the selection of a name for the child. The Tamil almanac (pañcankam) provides a set of initial syllables suitable for the child's astrological configuration, and a name is selected which begins with one of these syllables. Naming of children amongst the Moors is sometimes conditioned by numerological considerations and the advice of religious experts.

Brenda Beck reports from Coimbatore, Tamilnadu, that pregnant women are considered to be in a "heated condition" as a consequence of the accumulation of blood in the womb (1969, p. 562). Actually, none of my informants said so, but the existence of this cultural assumption can be inferred both from the indigenous theory of gestation and from the postnatal rules governing the care of the mother. Never having witnessed an actual birth scene in Batticaloa, I can only indicate what people said about the events surrounding the delivery. The new mother is generally not given food until the day following the birth, apparently because she is too exhausted. When she begins to take nourishment, she is first given *milakutannīr* ("pepper water", the British "mulligatawny soup"), a hot, pungent broth heavily spiced with chillies and extra amounts of garlic. These ingredients, especially chillies and garlic, are considered to be very "heating". Rice is often served in a mushy form (*kulaiyal*) which is considered easier to digest, accompanied by a curry made of one of the humourally "neutral" varieties of small lagoon fish (e.g. *cettal, varāl, kilakkan, mural, terali*). The new mother will be given coffee—heating, as opposed to tea, which is cooling—or at the very least hot water, to drink. In addition, some type of distilled alcoholic beverage, usually brandy or arrack, will be administered to the new mother daily on medicinal grounds as a tonic with strong "heating" qualities. One Ayurvedic specialist even offered the recipe for a special "arrack powder" (*cārāyaccūranam*) which is prescribed for postnatal mothers in distress. In short, there is a very strong emphasis on "heating" foods and substances in the postnatal diet, while at the same time, there is a strict prohibition on fruits (generally cooling), milk and yoghurt (cooling). There is explicit anxiety that the new mother may suffer "cool illnesses" (*kulir varuttam*), and this danger evidently arises from the abrupt loss of the mother's blood and bodily heat when the baby is born. There are at the same time other medical concerns, particularly the need to stop the bleeding and to promote the rapid healing of what are considered to be the wounds within the mother's womb. Milk and yoghurt are said to inhibit the healing of wounds, and to cause wind and indigestion; it was for these reasons, rather than their "cooling" quality, that most people forbade their consumption. At some point, the desire to generate "heat" within the mother's body must conflict with the desire to "cool" and heal her wounds, since heat agitates the blood and aggravates all open sores. The conventional compromise is to restrict the intake of some strong or heating foods, such as chicken, beef, or eggs, until the mother's condition has improved, while just as during the female puberty rite, an oral dose or two of margosa oil (extremely cooling) is administered to cool and heal the womb itself.[20]

The period of ritual pollution arising from childbirth lasts for 31 days among the Tamils and 40 days among the Moors, and it is within the framework of this pollution period that the special postnatal dietary and behavioral rules are applied. The birth pollution gradually lessens during this period, the health of the mother and child gradually improve, and the mother gradually returns to a normal diet. There is probably considerable variation in the timing of this transition, but after the twelfth day it is common for the mother to bathe with normal cool well water, rather than with special hot water. She can also begin to take more "cooling" foods, such as *taṉṉīrccōṟu* ("water-rice", cooked rice soaked in water, eaten with coconut milk and jaggary). Certain prohibitions, such as the rule against milk and yoghurt, are enforced throughout the entire pollution period, but my impression is that other dietary practices depend on the speed of the mother's recovery. That the twelfth day marks a customary transition out of the most polluting and most dangerous postnatal phase is also indicated by special payments of food for the household Washerman and the midwife on this day, which is called "twelfth rice".

Final Purifications, Protections and Practices

The end of the 31 days of childbirth pollution is marked in a Tamil home by a purification of the house, a ritual bath for the mother and the shaving of the child's head. Because this event is accompanied by domestic entertaining as well as by substantial payments of food, clothing and liquor to the household Washerman and Barber, it is sometimes called the "31st (day) expense" (*muppattiyōrāṉ celavu*). The mother's bath is merely a full "head bath" without much ritual elaboration. The tonsure of the infant is performed by the household Barber caste man, who also pierces the child's ears as a mark of Hindu religious identity. The removal of the child's hair is said to symbolically remove any ritual pollution still adhering to the child from its contact with the mother's vagina, but it is also a kind of sacrifice as well as a symbolic "new start" in life. On or around the 31st day, it is also customary to tie a heavy black thread around the child's waist. Males wear such a thread or silver chain, called an *aruṇā koṭi* (lit. *araiṉāṉ*, "waist string"), for the rest of their lives, while female children only wear it for a short while. After I got beyond the true, but inadequate, explanation that this thread holds up a man's underwear (*kaccai*, loincloth), everyone admitted that it was universally believed to give men "strength in the waist" (*iṭappil pelaṉ*). Typically, the overt reference was to physical strength to perform labour in the fields, but some people later admitted it included sexual vigour. Females do not wear the waist string because they possess an inherent excess of blood, *cakti*, and sexual desire already.

Among Moors, the end of ritual contamination on the 40th day is likewise marked by a bath for the mother and tonsure for the infant, but the latter will be performed by the hereditary Muslim barber/circumciser (*Ostā māmā*) or by a man of the household. If the infant is a girl, she will receive a visit from the barber/circumciser's wife (*Ostā māmi*) near the end of the 40 day period. Most of my informants said that she makes a tiny prick or incision in the baby's genitals sufficient to draw blood, but a few thought that the tip of the clitoris was actually severed. The truth is that most of these accounts came from males, who have no clear idea of what is actually done. My evidence indicates that present practice is no more than a symbolic mutilation carried out in the name of Islamic tradition, but several Moorish men also asserted the aim of the operation was to reduce (whether symbolically or surgically) the excessive sexual desire of women. The corresponding male circumcision among Moors does not take place until the boy is nine or ten years old.

Lactation: Milk from Blood

The beginning of lactation is recognized to entail some pain in the breasts (*pāl nōkkāṭu, pāl vētaṇai,* "milk pains"), and the colostrum itself is called "throbbing milk" (*kaṭuppuppāl*). The standard belief is that the colostrum is a weak or impure form of milk, not suitable for the child to digest. Consequently, the infant may suckle primarily from a wet-nurse for the first three days, as well as enjoy jaggary suckers (*paṇaṅkuṭṭān*), while the mother manually draws off the colostrum. Breast milk is a product or transformation of the blood in the same way that semen is, although no standard ratio of blood to milk is cited. Two people even said that milk, like semen, forms in a semi-solid lump at the top of the head which subsequently "melts" and flows to the breasts during lactation. Traditional medical belief places great importance on the supply of mothers' milk, and one frequently hears the lament that today's women no longer have the lactational capacity of their forbears (hence the modern fall-back to bottle feeding). However, some of the very foods which are believed to promote lactation are restricted during the initial postnatal period on the grounds that they may hinder or delay the mother's healing. Milk and yoghurt are often mentioned as being specifically likely to promote lactation, but these are generally given only after the end of the childbirth pollution period. Coconut milk is considered generically equivalent to cow or buffalo milk, but less potent, so it may be given before dairy milk is permitted.

The commonly accepted opinion is that the baby should be weaned from the breast by nine months or a year, and a bitter substance such as margosa oil may be smeared on the nipples to encourage this. There is no standard period of postpartum taboo on sexual relations, but I doubt if anyone commencing intercourse before six months would admit it. Ideally, one should probably wait a year. Intimacy during the period of lactation, and contact with the wife's breasts or milk, posed a ritual danger to husbands in ancient Tamilnadu (Hart, 1973, pp. 234–236). Although I found no such belief in Batticaloa today, the breast is still an extraordinarily private and sacrosanct part of a fertile woman's body. The first solid foods given to the infant include rice flour pudding (kali) mixed with a bit of Ethiopian cumin (ōmam, acamatākam, L. Sison ammi) and jaggary, as well as mashed bananas. Later, the child will start taking mashed rice mixed with broth (racam). Even after weaning, the child's food is cooked and served by the mother's hands, so that the transfer of "maternal" substance, together with maternal affection, is seen to continue through childhood.

Influencing Fertility

As my description of the female puberty rituals alone might indicate, there is tremendous cultural emphasis upon the ideal of the woman as chaste wife and fertile mother. A newlywed couple lives matrilocally at least for a year or two, during which period they are given especially nourishing food, relieved of some of the more onerous domestic tasks and afforded extra rest and privacy. Some of this is justified as a gentle transition into new marital roles, but the other aim is clearly to encourage sexual relations and to get the wife pregnant as quickly as possible. In fact, as a consequence of their presumed coital obsession, the new couple are sometimes said to have a mild sort of ritual pollution which should keep them out of Hindu temples for the first six months of marriage. This is considered a small price to pay for quick offspring.

Strategies Against Barrenness

A wife without children is both personally unfulfilled and ritually inauspicious. Concern with problems of infertility is reflected in a pragmatic diversity of diagnostic and therapeutic strategies, some of which can be pursued simultaneously without contradiction. The basic assumption in Batticaloa, as throughout the South Asian culture area, is that infertility is primarily due to a problem with the woman. Beyond this, barrenness may be attributed to some supernatural agency, but seldom is the potency of the husband questioned. An infertile woman (*malaṭi*) who seeks treatment in the domain of traditional medicine is given standard assurances that "there is no such thing in the whole world as a truly barren woman" (*peṇmalaṭu ulakattil yārumillai*), but the diagnoses can sound fairly dire: destabilizing humours (windy, eruptive), blockage of the womb, diminished or contaminated blood supply, tiny organisms (*kirumi*) which eat the seminal fluids. For some (occasionally all) of these conditions there are complex herbal compounds which are prescribed according to instructions encoded in traditional medical songs. It is virtually impossible to elicit a quick, succinct summary of such medicines and their uses, because the songs are indespensible mnemonics and must be recited from the beginning each time.

The ingredients (*carakku*, medicinal substances) used in compounding fertility tonics are drawn from the traditional Ayurvedic pharmacopoeia, available from specialized herbal shops in all major towns, if not from the local environment itself. Most of the herbal compounds I recorded contained upwards of twenty ingredients, and without recourse to formal training in the Ayurvedic system I am unable to characterize the reasoning behind their efficacy beyond the general principle that excess bodily humours must be balanced and compensated. The chief etiology identifies certain classes of disorders (e.g. *vāta nōykaḷ*, "wind diseases"), any one of which may produce barrenness together with other symptoms. Consequently, medical verses for some of the more complex herbal compounds often read like a musical panacea.

When I asked about male sterility, the medical experts admitted it was possible, but they said that male patients never seek help and that most men would never acknowledge the possibility by accepting medication. Even so, there is an obvious concern with excess heat in the male body, a heat which is sometimes manifested in urinary and venereal disease (*mēkaviyāti, piramēkam*). The various types of venereal disease all involve the loss or contamination of male semen, either through uncontrolled "leaking", bleeding in the urinary tract, or thin, watery semen. The excess heat which produces such weakened semen may derive from any number of sources, including excessive sexual intercourse itself.[21] While this diagnosis suggests the need to cool the body and concentrate the semen through greater sexual abstinence, there can also be a quite different diagnosis for male sterility: insufficient libido. As a matter of fact, only a few preparations for male sterility were ever cited, but they all turned out to be exotic aphrodisiacs with names like *maṉmata ilēkiyam* ("Kāma's electuary") or *vīriya virutti paṇṇiraṇṭu* ("the semen-increasing twelve"). There are also foods which aid in the production of semen: honey, ghee, yoghurt (especially if it

has a thick rubbery crust), jaggary, meat and eggs. Many of these are refined or thickened substances with clear affinities to the admired qualities of semen itself. Finally, there are the everyday aphrodisiacs, raw onion and woodapple, said to incite seminal emissions so strongly that they are banned from the diet of students at the Ramakrishna Mission Hostel.

With barrenness carrying such a heavy stigma in this society, many infertile women have simultaneous recourse to ethno-medical and to supernatural cures. Despite the intricate ethno-medical theories of conception which I have outlined, there is a tendency to think of children as a gift of God. There is first of all the possibility that infertility, like some other afflictions, has been induced by the influence or presence of malevolent spirits acting independently or as agents of sorcery (*cūniyam*). Hence there is a chance that magical countermeasures undertaken through a friendly *mantiravāti* (lit. "reciter of mantras") will exorcise and dispel these spirits. It is just as likely, however, that a childless woman (or a childless couple) will make a vow (*nērttikkaṭan*) to a Hindu deity or to a local Muslim saint, a vow which attributes no divine blame for the lack of children, but which pledges fulfillment of a contractual agreement if the deity or saint grants the boon of fertility. Such vows can be made locally, but they are often fulfilled by pilgrimage to a larger regional shrine. Completion of such vows usually involves making food offerings (e.g. *pukkai*, sweetened milk-rice, later shared among the worshippers), but Hindus may also bring a miniature votive offering (*aṭaiyāḷam*, "symbolic representation"). The treasuries of Hindu temples accumulate a vast array of such offerings, usually made of silver, each typically the replica of an afflicted organ or a missing object, and perhaps the most common of such offerings is the *piḷḷaiyum toṭṭilum*, the tiny silver "child and cradle". Other simple offerings are rocks, each one brought by a childless couple, heaped conspicuously atop hills associated with nearby Murugan temples. The most popular deities for making fertility vows are Piḷḷaiyār (Ganesh), Murugaṉ (Kataragama) and Kaṇṇaki (the Sinhalese Pattini), but such vows are probably made to all deities. However, in Batticaloa, the cult of the cobra god Nākatampirāṉ, while extremely popular as protection against snakebite, lacks the strong association with fertility and gynaecological problems it has in Jaffna (Pfaffenberger, 1977).

Contraception: Traditional and Modern

In the past few years, the rate of population growth in Sri Lanka has shown a significant decline, although the contribution of government-sponsored contraception programmes to this has probably had less importance than a general rise in the marriage age of women. In any event, the rate of contraceptive use in most parts of Batticaloa at this time is still quite low, particularly among the semi-urban Moors and the rural Tamils. A survey questionnaire carried out in 1974 reveals that when "natural" methods such as abstinence, rhythm method and coital withdrawal are included, upwards of 40% of married couples can be said to use some birth control technique, but actually only 7% use any contraceptive device. Another 40% of the sample were currently non-users but indicated a desire to use some method of contraception in the future, yet most of these people are probably contemplating only "natural" methods (Population Services International, 1974).[22] While my research indicates that many people are worried that the pill (the most common of the artificial birth control methods) poses a danger to a woman's health,[23] the "natural" methods are largely in accord with traditional values of self-restraint, conservation of semen and avoidance of pollution, as well as with the ideal of spacing births. The health of the mother is one goal in the spacing of births, and another goal is the establishment of a clear age hierarchy among siblings. Relative age is a very important principle of social authority and deference which is also systematically expressed in all of the Sri Lankan Dravidian-type kinship terminologies. Within a family, pressure for the parents to observe total sexual abstinence arises when the eldest daughters are given matrilocally in marriage: there is a cultural assumption that the locus of active sexuality should, at that point, pass to the next generation.

One contraceptive technique which has recently been promoted is the condom, marketed under the subsidized trademark PREETHI (Tamil and Sinhalese "bliss") in village-level boutiques and shops throughout the island. In discussions of the condom with my male informants, it became clear that its main practical drawback is the problem of disposal, while a latent ethnomedical problem is whether blocking male semen and placing a latex barrier between the partners will reduce the tangible somatic benefits of intercourse. The "benefits" in this case refer to the transfer of some vaguely identified blood or bodily essence between the sexual partners. Just as male blood (in the form of semen) goes into the female, some people felt that at least a tiny bit of female blood (or female semen) entered the man's penis during sex. Others could not specify exactly how the process occurs, but they felt that an older man, for example, receives some sort of invigorating influence from sex (in moderation, of course) with a young, healthy woman, whereas intercourse with an older woman can kill a younger man. An explanation of the latter belief is that individuals, although they lose blood in aging, nevertheless gain in bodily heat, "just as a pressure-lamp becomes hotter and hotter as the fuel is used up" (c.f. Tamilnadu data on aging, Beck, 1963, p. 562). An unfavourable balance of bodily heat is often cited as a cause of infertility and uro-genital disorders. On the other hand, the potential benefits for an older man of sex with a young woman must be balanced against the risks inherent in the diminution of his own blood and the loss of his vital semen. The belief that the blood or the "pulse" of the man and the woman is exchanged or mixed during coitus is apparently stronger and more explicit in the Sinhalese population (Kemper, 1979, pp. 488–489). I also learned from a Colombo-based family planning official that young Sinhalese men in some areas had openly voiced fears that use of the condom would deprive them of vital female blood.[24]

From the standpoint of formal religious doctrine, the Hindu Tamils in Batticaloa do not have a "position" on birth control, except that they uniformly abhor abortion. The Moors, on the other hand, can easily obtain sermons on the anti-Islamic nature of contraception from local Muslim religious experts. The Muslim position is quite similar to that of the second-largest monotheistic group in the Batticaloa region, the Roman Catholics: contraception subverts the divine purpose for sexual relations, which is to engender offspring. However, I have no reason to suppose that Muslims would be any more likely than Catholics to forswear contraception on religious grounds alone. An equally impor-tant "external" source of pressure for or against birth control pro-grammes is political sensitivity to demographic balances between the major ethnic/religious groups in the Sri Lankan population. For this reason, some of the more politically astute Batticaloa Moors are content to endorse the fundamentalist position that large families are the will of Allah. On the other hand, it is my impression that the politically disenfranchised Estate Tamil tea pickers have received the most effective vasectomy programme in the island.

Conclusions

This account of sexuality, fertility and childbirth in eastern Sri Lanka has been offered, not only for its ethnomedical interest, but also as a contribution to the analysis of regional variation in South Asia. The isolation of the Batticaloa region, its peripheral Tamil identity in relation to the dominant Sinhalese Buddhist culture of the island, its matrilineal social organization, and its own internal Hindu/Muslim multi-ethnicity would all seem to suggest considerable grounds for variation from pan-Indian cultural norms. However, elements of the traditional Ayurvedic humoural theory of medicine are clearly present, as well as some familiar South Asian beliefs about blood and its transformations. What this research reveals is that traditional ethnomedical theories may be given a reinterpretation, or at least a selective regional emphasis, to make them fit better with local cultural and social structural patterns. For example, some typical South Asian beliefs about the potency of male semen are found here, but the distinctive Batticaloa concern with matriliny and the "maternal connection" is incorporated into prevailing ethnomedical theory by special emphasis upon maternal blood transfusion in the womb and via the lactating breast. The bilateral aspects of conception, recognized to some extent in all South Asian medical theory, is expressed here more systematically, and with more attention to the female component, than in patrilineal areas of South Asia. At the same time, the cultural impact of patrilineal ideas from Jaffna and south India can be detected in the confused and divided opinions of some informants regarding the identity of the child's blood and the spread of death pollution. Finally, even in this matrilocal society, the common Indic symbols of male/female hierarchy are recognized, as theories of the sex of the embryo confirm.

Theories of ritual temperature and humoural balance in Batticaloa are broadly consistent with the growing literature on the "grammar" of South Asian ritual, i.e. the cultural assumptions which lie behind and, to a surprising extent, unify the logic of medicine, diet, and relations with the supernatural. The explanation of blood as the quintessence of bodily strength, the belief that it can be transformed into refined bodily essences (milk, semen), the associations between blood and heat, power and sexual control—these are all features of South Asian thought which inform, in a variety of local ways, both the meaning of health and the meaning of ritual. In Batticaloa, it has been shown that a common set of ethnomedical and ritual assumptions pervades both Hindu and Muslim daily life, despite ethnic and doctrinal conflicts on other levels. At the same time, it is ritual practice, rather than ethnomedical belief, which is more vulnerable to public pressure, as discontinuance of the Moorish girls' puberty ceremony seems to show.

Analysis of ethnomedical assumptions regarding puberty and reproductive processes illuminates the similarities and differences between first menstruation rites and childbirth practices. In puberty rites, the girl is "hot" because of excess blood which has accumulated in her body: she is therefore given "cooling" substances and foods. After giving birth, the mother's body is in danger of excessive "coolness" arising from the sudden departure of the child, whose body has been accumulating the mother's blood throughout gestation: she is therefore given "heating" substances and foods. In both cases, however, her womb is believed to have sustained wounds which must quickly be healed: she is therefore kept away from dairy products (which are cooling, but slow down healing) and *kiranti* foods (which are heating, but eruptive).

Concern with ritual pollution is a basic feature of female puberty rituals as well as childbirth practices. On these occasions one sees clearly how the Washerman and the Barber, the Midwife and the Circumciser, serve to perform the most polluting operations and to remove the influence of pollution from the domestic sphere. The status of these specialists is low, but recognition of the service they perform is constantly dramatized: custom demands they be given prescribed items of payment for their services at almost every stage of the ritual sequence. On the other hand, puberty and manhood rites among the Tamils and the Moors also show strong symbolic affinities to the wedding ritual (*kaliyāṇam*), the most pure and auspicious rite of passage. In addition to the various ethnomedical presuppositions which have already been discussed, these rituals also presuppose the active involvement of real or classificatory cross-kin, who are affines and preferred marriage partners.

When attention is turned to problems of infertility, one immediately sees the importance of pluralistic systems of diagnosis and cure. Cures for barrenness may be sought through traditional folk medicine, exorcism techniques and vows to deities and saints. Precautions may also be taken against astrological factors, the evil eye, and inauspicious sights. While there are important symbolic connections between these levels of belief, the individual exercises great pragmatic discretion in the choice of diagnosis and treatment. No standard hierarchy of recourse to treatment seems to exist, and patients often pursue more than one sort of cure at the same time.

Finally, traditional ideas about birth control in Batticaloa reflect fundamental concerns with sexual control, the containment of pollution, the promotion of the mother's health and the spacing of births. There is clear scope for modern birth control programmes within these basic values, but birth control agencies might acquire greater sensitivity to variations in underlying ethnomedical beliefs, and gain access to a wider constituency, by training non-Western curing practitioners to dispense contraceptive information and materials (Taylor, 1976).

Acknowledgements

I am grateful for the research support provided by U.S. Public Health Service NIMH Predoctoral Fellowship no. MH38122 and Research Grant no. MH11765, British SSRC research grants no. HR5549/1 and 2, the Smuts Memorial Fund and the Travelling Expenses Fund of Cambridge University, and the Andrew Mellon Postdoctoral Fellowship Program of Cornell University. I would also like to express my appreciation to George L. Hart for his assistance with Tamil poetry and to K. Kanthanathan, V. Ratnam, Nilam Hamead and K. Mahesvaralingam for their contributions to the fieldwork.

Notes

(1) For an introduction to the literature on Ayurveda see Leslie (1976). Actually, some of my practitioner-informants referred to their medical system as *cittāyulvētam,* raising at least the possibility of a connection with the south Indian Tamil Siddha (*cittar*) yogico-medical tradition (Zvelebil, 1973). However, the only tangible evidence of this I ever came across was a reference to an ethno-chemical theory of "male" salts and "female" acids (see the section on The Reproductive Process and Note 13).

(2) Muslim curing practitioners in the Batticaloa region do not participate in a distinctive or separate Muslim medical tradition, such as Ūnāni (Leslie, 1976). In fact, one local Muslim specialist assured me that the medical knowledge which had come to him through his forefathers had originated with Lord Civa. The views represented in this study are primarily those of high caste Hindu males. A quarter (9/35) of these, including two Moors, were full or part-time non-Western curing practitioners; a handful (4/35) were Vīracaiva Kurukkaḷ temple priests; a similar number (6/35) were low caste informants (1 Smith, 1 Washerman, 4 Paṟaiyar Drummers). Of necessity, my female informants were primarily the wives and mothers of my closest acquaintances. Not every person with whom I spoke could answer all the specialized questions I asked, but the sample consisted of the most knowledgeable people in these areas of inquiry. The data they supplied has the characteristic strengths and weaknesses of all intensive first-hand fieldwork data, but I think the most important potential sources of bias have been mentioned.

(3) I could find no support in my research for the contention by Marriott and Inden (1977) and Marriott (1976) that traditional South Asian medical doctrines rationalize an entire theory of caste society, any more than Dumont's (1970) emphasis upon the "religion of pure and impure" could be seen to encompass them.

(4) At this point an astute local critic spotted an awkward contradiction between traditional diagnosis and Western medicine: if the elderly have such weakened force of blood, why do government doctors report so many of them dying of "high blood pressure"?

(5) In colloquial Tamil, *camaiccāccu*. Beck has pointed out that the verb *camai* in its transitive form means "to cook" and in its intransitive form means "to mature" (Beck, 1969, p. 562).

(6) Deborah Winslow (1980) has pointed out some of the uniformities of first menstruation rituals throughout Sri Lanka. Nur Yalman has offered a lengthy analysis of the significance of the Sinhalese girls' puberty rite (Yalman, 1963).

(7) Rev. Miron Winslow (1862, p. 300) associates *kiranti* with venereal ulcers, which is also consistent with the concern to heal the girl's womb after the first menstruation.

(8) A similar practice is reported in the Nayar rite of first menstruation, *tirandukuli* (Puthenkalam, 1977, p. 59).

(9) As Beck has noted, milk and fruit are "cooling" substances which would help to offset the "heating" effects of post-nuptial coitus (1969, p. 564).

(10) There is a reference to this ceremony in Simon Casie Chitty's *Ceylon Gazetteer* (1834, pp. 245–247, 279–80), where the youth is said to be shaved with milk.

(11) The common word for the Muslim circumcision in this region is *cuṇṇattu* (Arabic *sunnat*, custom sanctioned by the Prophet), but on printed invitations it is sometimes given the loftier Sanskritic title of *viruttacētaṇam*, "maturity cutting".

(12) The testicles, although mentioned as a conduit for semen, were not thought to be the fundament of male sexuality. Their practical importance is recognized in the gelding of bullocks, but this was explained to me as forcing upon the beast a sort of artificial asceticism which redirects its semen into forms of bodily strength (and by implication, spiritual docility).

(13) Rev. Miron Winslow (1862, p. 411). This type of ethno-chemical classification is characteristic of the Tamil Siddha medical and yogic system (Zvelebil, 1973, p. 32, Note 31; p. 36, Note 44).

(14) Compare this with Koṇṭaikkaṭṭi Vēḷāḷar beliefs in Tamilnadu: "KVs say father's blood gives a child form or body (*uṭampu*) and mother's blood gives a child motion or spirit (*uyir*)" (Barnett, 1976, p. 146).

(15) The umbilical cord is said to develop only at a late stage in the growth of the foetus. Its purpose is to carry liquified food (chyme) to the foetus when direct transfusion of blood is no longer required. The fact that traditional medicine is a male profession, yet men never lay eyes on a placenta or an umbilical cord, may have some-

thing to do with the de-emphasis of the umbilical connection in medical lore.

(16) Both among the Kandyan Sinhalese (Yalman, 1967, p. 137) and among Koṇṭaikkaṭṭi Vēḷāḷars in Tamilnadu (Barnett, 1976, p. 146) it is reported that repeated sexual intercourse is recommended during pregnancy to supply additional male semen which will nourish or strengthen the foetus. One term for the heat generated in sexual intercourse in the Batticaloa region is *akkaṟaiccūṭu* ("heat of urgency"). It poses a threat of colic and digestive disorders (*māntam*) in the newborn infant.

(17) Aside from these medical songs, many informants volunteered the opening lines from the 15th century poem, *Uṭaṟkūṟṟuvaṇṇam*, by the Tamil Siddha poet Paṭṭiṇattār, which traces the human body from conception, through maturation, to ultimate decay. The poem has been translated by Zvelebil (1973, pp. 102–107).

(18) In south India and in Tamil areas of Sri Lanka, the Barber serves as the funeral priest. Perhaps because of this inauspicious association with death, the role of midwife in Batticaloa is more often identified with the Washerman caste. Barber midwives are not unknown, but my data do not completely support Thurston's comment that Barbers are "the recognized midwives of the Hindu community in the Tamil country" (Thurston, 1909, p. 32).

(19) I was told that in the old days, when clocks were not available, someone would immediately sever the trunk of a plantain tree: the exact time of birth could be deduced the next day by examining the growth of the innermost part of the stalk.

(20) In some cases, a belief in the universal efficacy of margosa oil may outweigh the consideration of its specific humoural value in treating a patient. Margosa oil is so highly esteemed that it is sometimes referred to as *taṇi eṇṇey*, "the only oil".

(21) Much of what local specialists said about male semen diseases fits theoretically with what Obeyesekere has reported from Sinhalese areas (1976, pp. 207–215). However, the level of popular anxiety about this in Batticaloa seems to be much lower. I only heard *piramēkam* discussed by Ayurvedic specialists, and rarely at that.

(22) One of the most ingenious local theories about "natural" contraception I encountered was put forth by a Tamil clerk who had spent some time pondering the commonly accepted view that Moors produce more children than Tamils. It is widely thought that the Muslim consumption of beef (an extremely "hot" form of meat) enhances their sexual power. However, this man also drew attention to the circumcision of Moorish men, contending that it results in a desensitization of the penis sufficient to prolong

intercourse, thereby making female orgasm more likely. Since female semen and male semen must be ejaculated simultaneously if the chances of impregnation are to be maximized, this would explain the higher Moorish fertility.

(23) This fear is not unreasonable, given the arbitrary dosages and fluctuating supplies of birth control pills in some localities.

(24) The inverse concern is reported amongst the Koṇṭaikkaṭṭi Vēḷāḷars of Tamilnadu, who fear that polluted blood might enter a man's penis and mix with his own blood during intercourse with a low caste woman (Barnett, 1976, p. 144).

References

Babb, L. A. (1975). *The Divine Hierarchy: Popular Hinduism in Central India.* New York: Columbia University Press.

Banks, M. Y. (1957). The social organization of the Jaffna Tamils of North Ceylon, with special reference to kinship, marriage, and inheritance. Unpublished Ph.D. thesis, Cambridge University.

Barnett, S. A. (1976). "Cocoanuts and Gold: Relational Identity in a South Indian Caste". *Contributions to Indian Sociology* N.S. **10** (1), 133–156.

Beck, B. E. F. (1969). "Colour and Heat in South Indian Ritual". *Man* N.S. **4**, 553–572.

Carstairs, G. M. (1957). *The Twice Born: A Study of a Community of High Caste Hindus.* London: Hogarth Press.

Casie Chitty, S. (1834). *The Ceylon Gazetteer.* Ceylon: Cotta Church Mission Press.

David, K. (1973). "Until Marriage Do Us Part: A Cultural Account of Jaffna Tamil Categories for Kinsmen". *Man* N.S. **8**, 521–535.

Douglas, M. (1966). *Purity and Danger: An Analysis of Concepts of Pollution and Taboo.* London: Routledge and Kegan Paul.

Dube, L. (1978). The Seed and the Earth: Symbolism of Human Reproduction in India. Paper presented at 10th International Congress of Anthropological and Ethnological Sciences. New Delhi, December 1978.

Dumont, L. (1970). *Homo Hierarchicus: The Caste System and its Implications.* Chicago: University of Chicago Press.

Fruzzetti, L. and Östör, A. (1976). "Seed and Earth: A Cultural Analysis of Kinship in a Bengali Town". *Contributions to Indian Sociology* N.S. **10** (1), 97–132.

Hart, G. L., III (1973). "Women and the Sacred in Ancient Tamilnad". *Journal of Asian Studies* **32**, 233–250.

Kemper, S. E. G. (1979). "Sinhalese Astrology, South Asian Caste Systems, and the Notion of Individuality". *Journal of Asian Studies* **38**, 477–497.

Leach, E. R. (1961). *Pul Eliya, a Village in Ceylon: A Study of Land Tenure and Kinship.* Cambridge: Cambridge University Press.

Leslie, C. M. (ed.) (1976). *Asian Medical Systems: A Comparative Study.* Berkeley: University of California Press.

Manu (G. Bühler, trans.) (1886). *The Laws of Manu.* Oxford: Clarendon Press.

Marriott, McK. (1976). "Hindu Transactions: Diversity Without Dualism". In *Transactions and Meaning: Directions in the Anthropology of Exchange and Symbolic Behavior* (B. Kapferer, ed.), pp. 109–142. Philadelphia: Institute for the Study of Human Issues.

Marriott, McK. and Inden, R. (1977). "Toward an Ethnosociology of South Asian Caste Systems". In *The New Wind: Changing Identities in South Asia* (K. David, ed.), pp. 226–238. The Hague: Mouton.

Mayer, A. C. (1960). *Caste and Kinship in Central India: A Village and its Region.* Berkeley: University of California Press.

McGilvray, D. B. (1973). "Caste and Matriclan Structure in Eastern Sri Lanka: A Preliminary Report on Fieldwork in Akkaraipattu". *Modern Ceylon Studies* **4**, 5–20.

McGilvray, D. B. (1974). Tamils and Moors: caste and matriclan structure in eastern Sri Lanka. Unpublished Ph.D. thesis, University of Chicago.

McGilvray, D. B. (ed.) (in press). "Mukkuvar Vannimai: Tamil Caste and Matriclan Ideology in Batticaloa, Sri Lanka". In *Caste Ideology and Interaction.* Cambridge: Cambridge University Press.

Obeyesekere, G. (1963). "Pregnancy Cravings (*dola-duka*) in Relation to Social Structure and Personality in a Sinhalese Village". *American Anthropologist* **65**, 323–342.

Obeyesekere, G. (1967). *Land Tenure in Village Ceylon.* Cambridge: Cambridge University Press.

Obeyesekere, G. (1976). "The Impact of Āyurvedic Ideas on the Culture and the Individual in Sri Lanka". In *Asian Medical Systems: a Comparative Study* (C. M. Leslie, ed.), pp. 201–226. Berkeley: University of California Press.

O'Flaherty, W. D. (1969). "Asceticism and Sexuality in the Mythology of Siva". *History of Religions* **8**, 300–337 and **9**, 1–41.

Pfaffenberger, B. L. (1977). Pilgrimage and traditional authority in Tamil Sri Lanka. Unpublished Ph.D. thesis, University of California.

Population Services International (1973). A survey of female family planning knowledge, attitudes and practices: Batticaloa administrative district. (Draft copy). Colombo: Marketing Research Department of Lever Brothers (Ceylon) Ltd., for Population Services International.

Puthenkalam, Fr. J., S. J. (1977). *Marriage and Family in Kerala, with Special Reference to Matrilineal Castes.* Calgary: Journal of Comparative Family Studies monograph series.

Taylor, C. E. (1976). "The Place of Indigenous Medical Practitioners in the Modernization of Health Services". In *Asian Medical Systems: a Comparative Study* (C. M. Leslie, ed.), pp. 285–299. Berkeley: University of California Press.

Thurston, E. (1909). *Castes and Tribes of Southern India.* Vol. I. Madras: Government Press.

Winslow, D. (1980). "Rituals of First Menstruation in Sri Lanka". *Man* N.S. **15**, 603–625.

Winslow, Rev. M. (1862). *A Comprehensive Tamil and English Dictionary of High and Low Tamil.* Madras: American Mission Press.

Yalman, N. (1963). "On the Purity of Women in the Castes of Ceylon and Malabar". *Journal of the Royal Anthropological Institute* **93**, 25–58.

Yalman, N. (1967). *Under the Bo Tree: Studies in Caste, Kinship, and Marriage in the Interior of Ceylon.* Berkeley: University of California Press.

Zvelebil, K. V. (1973). *The Poets of the Powers.* London: Rider & Co.

3. Enga Birth, Maturation and Survival: Physiological Characteristics of the Life Cycle in the New Guinea Highlands

B. M. GRAY

The quest for health, the attainment of adulthood, fertility and longevity is a constant theme of Yandapu Enga ritual and myth.[1] This is not to say that these are the sole interests expressed in ritual but simply that they are always of importance both in the aims and in the symbolic content of certain rites which the Enga believe to be central to their culture.

In order to establish the validity or otherwise of indigenous statements in regard to what appeared to be an expression of perceptions, this chapter will consist in part of a brief review of the medical literature on rates and patterns of infant mortality, maturation, aging and adult mortality in pretechnological societies, and in particular in New Guinea. Arguments on the efficaciousness or otherwise of certain of the actions to be described below will not be entered into. Of those practices in Enga society which are believed to maintain physical well-being, some are efficacious in the sense usually meant in the developed world, that is in preventing or ameliorating perceived physical difficulties, some appear to have no effect, while others may be positively harmful. I shall not enter into a discussion on the nature of causal relationships which may or may not hold between the physiological patterns, such as late puberty, relatively early menopause and high child mortality, common to many New Guinea societies, or the existence or non-existence of particular social institutions, such as initiation or puberty ritual, and various forms of genital operations. However, an understanding of the physiological reality common to almost all Melanesian societies, although it may not explain the great differences in emphasis on, for example, puberty rites and the separation of the sexes from area to area, it does provide a basis from which common themes appear to emerge. My aim will be simply to establish the validity of indigenous perceptions of the quality of life upon which certain expectations, and in some cases, actions, are based.

The 25 000 Yandapu Enga of the western highlands of New Guinea live in and around the Wabag valley. Yandapu Enga society, language and material culture were, in 1969 and 1970, when I was carrying out my research, very similar to Meggitt's description of the Mae Enga, who live about 30 miles to the east (Meggitt, 1965). All references to the Yandapu in this paper describe conditions as they were during those two years. The Yandapu Enga came under colonial administration only 15 years prior to this field work. They form part of the population of the Lagaip sub-district, which varies in altitude from between 7000 feet above sea level to 9000 feet. The population density averages from between 30 to 48 persons per square mile, spread over extremely rough terrain.

Enga Health Practices and Beliefs

The Yandapu Enga have little knowledge of the pharmacological value of herbs even though they are frequently used as symbolic objects in healing rituals. There is a good understanding of anatomy, due to the practice of carrying out autopsies in order to ascertain, not so much the physiological cause of death, but which malevolent spirit, or still living person, has willed that a particular person should die, and from which group compensation should be sought. An operation is also performed on the living whereby an infected pleural cavity is drained following, for instance, an arrow wound. There is also some understanding that certain diseases can be transmitted by personal contact.

The main concerns of this society, however, are the survival of infants, the attainment of maturity, the maintenance of health and well-being during adulthood and the prevention of various syndromes which the western observer would refer to as part of the process of aging. None of these are ever phrased in terms of disease prevention, since concepts of disease and aging as we know them have little place in

Enga thought, which emphasizes instead an opposition of various kinds of strengths and weaknesses.

For example, the Enga believe that long postpartum abstinence is necessary if infants are to survive, that boys must undergo puberty rites if they are to reach physiological maturity, that the attainment of male maturity is in some way an uncertain process and that the sexes must live separately both in order to make boys into men, and to prevent men from becoming weak and useless.[2]

Prolonged postpartum abstinence is maintained for two years or more, during which time infants are breast fed. When very young, infants are carried in net bags on the mother's back. It is difficult to say exactly how frequently they are fed during the day, since very young babies may not be looked at by men, and especially not by fathers, for fear of the war magic in which men must participate. Accidental exposure to the gaze of a man who has "strong" war magic is believed to kill the new born. Young infants are fed in the women's houses or in the gardens where women spend most of each day and stay in the net bag on the mother's back while she works. If the day is warm and dry, the bag is hung from a convenient branch.

Small babies sleep with the mother on her breast and are suckled throughout the night. When allowed to sleep on the breast in this way, the sucking reflex is activated every few minutes, except when the infant is deeply asleep.

As soon as they are physically able to do so, older infants are carried on their mother's shoulders. At this stage they are considered to be strong enough to withstand contact with adult men. They are fed on demand during the day, clinging as the mother walks and feeding at will whenever she sits down. They also sleep on the breast at night.

The Enga believe that a baby will die should the parents cohabit, because it may drink the father's war magic with its mother's milk. The father's semen is believed to be a potent source of his war magic, and it is said to mingle with the mother's milk within her body, thus constituting a grave danger to the suckling infant.[3] Furthermore, they believe that if postpartum abstinence is not maintained during lactation, not only will the feeding infant die, so too will the next born. It is said to be killed by the malevolent and jealous spirit of the dead elder child. In this way, parents who do not abstain until they have fully weaned a child may be punished by it for their neglect.

The Enga also believe that loss of weight together with general weakness and greying hair is a feminine condition, and specifically say that women display these characteristics and die earlier than do men. This is a common theme in both myth and ritual (see also Posala, 1969, p. 92). Prohibitions on contact between the sexes were therefore explained as attempts by men to avoid these afflictions and even death itself. (For a discussion of Enga sexual symbolism, see Gray, 1973, pp. 125–30 and 227–246).

The proscriptions which separate the sexes, and especially those of a ritual nature which operate during the bachelor rites to enable boys to attain manhood and invulnerability to injury, illness and aging, are said by the Enga to be the foundation upon which the whole of their culture is based. Many anthropologists who have worked in other parts of New Guinea report that a commonly stated aim of the ritual and social separation of the sexes, including menstrual prohibitions and puberty rites, is to enable men to avoid the afflictions of weakness, aging and early death, which the Enga at least believe to be inevitable in women, but avoidable in men. Similar statements have been recorded both in areas where the separation of the sexes reaches an extreme, with elaborate puberty ritual and male circumcision, and in other areas where sexual avoidances, although present, are less pronounced.

An understanding of the physiological realities which are part of daily existence in New Guinea may provide insights into this wide range of practices and beliefs, even if they do not explain their existence. They may well be consistent with physical patterns and events often found in developing countries, but no longer seen in the West. Since they are given by the people as the *raison d'être* for so many of their actions, it seems important to evaluate the physical validity of this set of ideas before considering its implication at any other level of enquiry. It seems reasonable to seek an empirical foundation for the beliefs that the Enga and many other groups have that (1) if parents resume sexual intercourse while an infant is still being breast-fed, the risk of it and any subsequent child dying is substantially increased; (2) that the onset of puberty is delayed and that pubescence is a prolonged, unsure process; (3) that women as well as being weaker than men, also age and die prematurely relative to men. Can these patterns, if they exist, be so overt that they could be readily observable to a given society, so that, for example, weakness, premature aging and an early death could easily be typified by that society as peculiarly female states of being? In the following sections of this paper, I shall argue that there is evidence that these biological patterns exist and that until quite recently they probably would have been observable within each generation to adult members of many New Guinea societies.

Epidemiological and Demographic Data on Infant and Child Mortality, Maturation, Aging and Adult Mortality in New Guinea

Studies are available which provide information on the survival of infants and children, the age at puberty and sex differentials in the rates of aging and mortality among adults in New Guinea. Data now available are relatively recent and may not fully reflect the traditional or pre-contact situation, since it is reasonable to assume, and there is demographic evidence to show, that health conditions today are better than before European contact. It is seldom possible to obtain quantitative evidence on truly "traditional" situations, as most of the data are from societies with some contact, even if only marginal, with western technology, especially medical technology. Mortality rates observed today are less than they would have been in the pre-contact situation. The rate of natural increase in New Guinea today is probably approaching 3% per annum; this implies a doubling of the population every 30 years. Given the sparseness of the population observed on contact and the nature of traditional land and food resources, sustained rates of natural increase of this magnitude would not have been possible (Biersteker, 1961; Van de Kaa, 1967; Scragg, 1957, 1969; Malcolm, 1969; Sturt, 1972).[4] On the other hand, contemporary patterns of morbidity and the kinds of diseases which afflict people today are probably similar to those of the past, even though in many areas rates of mortality may have declined.[5]

Despite these and other reservations to be discussed below, the biomedical and demographic data can provide a picture which is of importance to the anthropologist, since they reflect the biological reality of the whole life cycle, from birth to death, which is not easily observed in any society without recourse to quantitative data. They also give some idea of the pre-contact situation.

Some Medical Evidence in Support of Traditional Arguments for the Necessity of Prolonged Postpartum Abstinence in New Guinea

Under pre-contact circumstances in New Guinea, infant and early childhood mortality was high. The figures given vary from between 167 per 1000 to 350 per 1000 births under one year in West Iran during the

1940s and 1950s (Van de Kaa, 1967, table 1, p. 90; Biersteker, 1961, p. 11) to much lower rates more recently in other areas of Papua New Guinea.

High death rates under one year indicate a population which is barely replacing itself, since high infant mortality rates (i.e. deaths under one year) frequently are associated with high mortality in the one to five year age group (Dyson, 1977, p. 282). Scragg (1957, appendix C, p. 132) estimated that 300 per 1000 children born died by the age of five years in New Ireland during the period between 1928 and 1953. Malcolm (1969) reported that about 200 per 1000 of children born to the Bundi died by the age of five in 1958. In 1969, an estimate of about 240 per 1000 was made for the Lumi (Wark and Malcolm, 1969, p. 129). Buchbinder (1973) also recorded very high figures for the Maring. Before contact, mortality rates were probably equally high, as rates of natural increase appear to have been very low.

By 1967, Van de Kaa was able to report declines in infant mortality in Western New Guinea. Malcolm and Scragg independently also published material relating to declines in the Bundi population and other rural areas in 1969. Sturt, in 1972, reported a halving of infant mortality rates within a decade in the Sepik. All of the researchers favoured the introduction of medical services as the major reason for these rapid declines in mortality. (Bailey, 1963b, p. 10; Van de Kaa, 1967, p. 89; Malcolm, 1969, pp. 13–18; Malcolm, 1970, p. 19; Scragg, 1969, pp. 73–90; for contemporary world figures on infant mortality see Vallin, 1976).

Among the peoples of the far Western Highlands Sinnett (1977) reports a figure of 85 per 1000 children dying under the age of one year for the Enga clan of Murapin, and 74 per 1000 for the Baiyer River (Becroft et al., 1969). But he points out that these figures are considerably lower than the rate of 123.7 per 1000 reported by Vines for the Highlands in 1970 in his New Guinea Survey (Vines, 1970, p. 50). However, 42.8% of all Enga children in Sinnett's study died before they had reached "marriageable age". This figure is comparable to the high childhood mortality rates reported for many other Third World countries (Dyson, 1977).[6]

There was evidence of high infant mortality for the clan of *Menge*, the Enga group with whom I worked, and who were immediate neighbours of the Murapin and intermarried with them. In spite of a reluctance to mention the dead, women often said that they had given birth to children who had died in infancy and that this was a common experience. Many women said they had had as many die as survive, and a few had no surviving children after giving birth to as many as eight. These observations taken together with Sinnett's data suggest that, until recently, Enga infant and child mortality was substantially higher than it is today.

Postpartum Abstinence

There is a complex relationship between breast-feeding, spacing between births, the survival of children and customary proscriptions on postpartum cohabitation found in many societies. In order to gain some understanding of this relationship the following factors have to be considered. First, the necessity of breast-feeding for the survival of infants in the absence of adequate or suitable infant foods in order to avoid the risk of malnutrition and infection; secondly, the effect of pregnancy on lactation; thirdly, the relative unreliability of lactational amenorrhoea in reducing the risk of pregnancy; fourthly, the effect of short birth intervals on infant mortality. These points require discussion.

Postpartum Abstinence and the Necessity for Breastfeeding

In societies where there are no safe and sterile high protein and calorie "baby foods" available to mothers, there is no alternative to prolonged breast-feeding. Early weaning under traditional circumstances frequently leads to infant death. In New Guinea and in similar areas where dairy products or other highly concentrated protein and energy foods are not produced as a staple, suitable weaning diets are not available. The normal constituents of the Enga diet, especially the sweet potato, are low both in protein and in calories (Bailey, 1963a, p. 390; Jelliffe and Maddocks, 1964), and in order to obtain sufficient nutrients, an individual must consume very large quantities of food per day. The bulk of food required is often in excess of the capacity of very young children, and malnutrition commonly results from the child's inability to consume sufficient food rather than from the unavailability of food *per se*. This situation has been well documented (Nichol, 1971, pp. 83–88; Frood *et al.*, 1971). Therefore, due to the absence of a suitable low bulk supplementary diet, children in many parts of the world must be maintained on the breast for prolonged periods.

In many Third World societies, and in the New Guinea highlands, where there is no suitable alternative infant diet, no sterilizable cooking or feeding utensils and where pre-mastication by the mother may be the only means of preparing soft infant foods, early weaning from the breast is associated with frequent diarrhoea (Scrimshaw *et al.*, 1968, pp. 233–235). Indeed in this situation, infants not breast-fed may have an almost 100% mortality (Van Zijl, 1966, p. 261).[7]

A recent study in Gambia has shown that even the normal and necessary process of introducing supplementary foods in addition to breast milk for infants at about six months is, under these circumstances, associated with an increased incidence of diarrhoea so that the average infant may be ill for 20% of each month despite continued breast-feeding (Rowland *et al.*, 1978, pp. 136–138; see also Van Zjil, 1966).

It is generally accepted that there is a synergetic interaction between nutrition and infection, which may lead to frank malnutrition and death in a previously merely undernourished child. The immunological response to infection is impaired by malnutrition, rendering the human host more susceptible to further infection. For example, frequent diarrhoea and the loss of appetite often associated with illness can decrease nutritional resources. This can lead to further impairment of the immune response and increase the frequency and severity of subsequent infections (Scrimshaw *et al.*, 1968, pp. 249–251; Morley, 1973, pp. 180–184; Puffer and Serrano, 1973, p. 18; Schonland, 1973; Srikantia *et al.*, 1976; Nutrition Reviews, 1972; Sinnett, 1977, p. 74; Editorial, Papua and New Guinea Medical Journal, 1969, pp. 71–72).

Even the diarrhoea associated with normal supplementary feeding can lead to undernutrition, and can impair an infant's resistance to recurrent gastro-intestinal and upper respiratory tract infections. These, and not the more exotic diseases, are the two most common causes of child mortality in the developing world (Dyson, 1977, pp. 282–311). In New Guinea, nutritional status, and in its turn, resistance to disease, is further undermined by the widespread problem of infestation by intestinal parasites such as ascaris and hookworm, and to a lesser extent by malaria. These parasitic diseases reduce nutritional reserves and cause, as well as exasercbating anaemia, a universal problem throughout New Guinea in women of child-bearing age, in the new-born and in children generally (Editorial, Papua New Guinea Medical Journal, 1955–1956, p. 33; Drover and Maddocks, 1975, pp. 15–17; Crane and Kelly, 1972, p. 234; Stanhope, 1975).

The circumstances under which the Enga traditionally live (i.e. no suitable alternative infant diet and no sterilizable cooking nor feeding utensils) are similar to those described above where infants not breast-fed may have an almost 100% mortality rate. Enga observations of, and concern about, high infant mortality rates in nonbreast-fed babies is expressed in many ways. Under traditional circumstances, should a lactating mother die, her unweaned infant is placed alive in the grave with her. It is mourned with her, and considered already dead (see also Hogbin, 1943, p. 295). Orphans are not suckled by other lactating women, as the Enga emphatically believe that no woman could have enough milk to support two children for the required two or more years, and that to try to do so would risk the lives of both infants.[8]

Because of this strongly held belief, when twins were born, traditionally one (and not always the female) was left to die or was killed, so that at least one would survive. Stories were often told of how, in the past, an animal or spirit would sometimes save the life of an abandoned twin, who would then return to its parents later in life bringing them wealth and forgiveness. These tales seemed to me to express the unhappiness and sense of wrong-doing felt by parents who believed that they had no alternative, but to kill one child in order that another might survive.[9]

Even today, with the availability of western medical services it is difficult to maintain twins or infants who are not breast-fed either because of maternal lactational failure or maternal death. In Laiagam, the survival of twins frequently requires prolonged hospitalization of the mother and the babies in order to ensure that they receive sufficient sterile supplementary food. This means complete disruption of the mother's very important economic role, unless she is fortunate enough to have her house and gardens within a very short distance of the hospital.

Even women who have lost a child and have still retained lactation will not foster and breast-feed an unweaned orphan, as this would necessitate an adherance to the rule of postpartum abstinence for a child who could not necessarily be claimed as their own by the husband and the husband's patriclan. Fostering can occur where the bereaved mother is the wife of the same clan as the orphaned infant, but since the patriclan is a relatively small group, only rarely can a bereaved woman and an orphaned child be quickly brought together in this way.[10]

The Enga make a connection between the acceptance of food by infants from anyone other than the mother, and the development of vomiting and diarrhoea. These afflictions are believed to be caused by the hidden envy or *yama*[11] of those who see and admire a healthy infant. It is believed to pass from the hand of the giver, through his or her middle finger into the offered food, which when eaten by the child causes it to sicken with diarrhoea, and possibly to die. People are also careful not to compliment a mother on a healthy child, for fear this may indicate envy on their part. Neither do they offer food to infants, for if the child were later to die of one of the many afflictions of early childhood, it may be thought that their hidden envy was the cause, intentionally or unintentionally. Hogbin also mentions that in Wogeo, no one but an infant's own mother should hold it or feed it for much the same reasons (Hogbin, 1943, p. 294). Such prohibitions on handling food for infants probably do, under the circumstances described, reduce the incidence of potentially fatal gastro-intestinal infections.

Prolonged Postpartum Abstinence: the Deleterious Effect of Pregnancy on Lactation

The deleterious effect of a supervening pregnancy on lactation, causing a drop in milk volume, eventual cessation of lactation and early weaning of the older child has been well documented (Scrimshaw *et al.*, 1968, pp. 233–235; Cantrelle and Leridon, 1971, pp. 524–525; Tyson *et al.*, 1976).

As we have seen, there are hazards associated with the normal weaning process; but if premature weaning occurs due to a supervening pregnancy, the risk of mortality may be substantially increased especially under the age of one year (Cantrelle and Leridon, 1971, p. 524) and significantly increased at older ages as well (Scrimshaw *et al.*, 1968, p. 252).[12]

The Necessity of Prolonged Postpartum Abstinence due to the Unreliability of Lactational Amenorrhoea in Preventing Conception

This point is closely interlinked with the preceding one. Although lactation provides some degree of contraceptive protection through the associated amenorrhoea, this effect diminishes with time, and in part depends upon the intensity of suckling.[13] Lactational amenorrhoea can vary from a mean of three months up to 18 months or more (Tyson *et al.*, 1976). It reduces, but does not abolish, the possibility of pregnancy. Therefore, strict postpartum abstinence for a least two years is necessary under traditional circumstances to ensure prevention of pregnancy and premature cessation of lactation since a supervening pregnancy will result in a decline of milk volume or cessation of lactation, and this may jeopardize the child's health by the introduction of unsafe weaning foods (Van Ginneken, 1974, pp. 201–206; Jain, 1977, pp. 1–34; Gopalan and Nadamuni Haidu, 1972).

Postpartum Abstinence: the Prevention of Short Birth Intervals and the Risk of Infant and Early Child Mortality

Short birth intervals are related to increased infant mortality, and this relationship is pronounced and present in all societies which have been studied (Hogbin, 1943, pp. 294–295; Morrison *et al.*, 1959; Wyon and Gordon, 1962, pp. 24–27; Wray, 1971, pp. 434–445; Addo and Goody, 1974; Wolfers and Scrimshaw, 1975; Omran and Standley, 1976, pp. 522–523). There is evidence to suggest that for many reasons, one infant death predisposes a family to subsequent child loss (Stoeckel and Chowdhury, 1972).

Premature conception and lactational failure are associated with high infant mortality of the first child. There is also an increased risk of death to the succeeding child born after a short birth interval, whether or not the elder child has survived (Wolfers and Scrimshaw, 1975). This risk is linked to factors such as reduced intensity of maternal care and to poor maternal nutritional status. For instance, short birth intervals can deplete maternal nutritional reserves, contributing to low birth weight and prematurity in the subsequent infant, which may lead to its death early in childhood (Venkatchalam, 1962, pp. 193–201; Wyon and Gordon, 1962; Wray and Aguirre, 1969; Wolfers and Scrimshaw, 1975). Furthermore, if a woman becomes pregnant again soon after the death of a preceding child, the drain on her nutritional resources increases, with the risk of the birth of an underweight baby, possible lactational failure and the eventual death of the subsequent infant (see the discussion below on maternal health).

The Enga belief that if a child is born before its preceding sibling had reached the usual age of weaning (i.e. between two and two and a half years), both children are likely to die, reflects clearly observable patterns of infant mortality in New Guinea. Short birth intervals in Enga society are largely caused by two factors: (a) conception which occurs while still breast-feeding, due to the breaking of the postpartum abstinence rule; (b) the death of a still breast-fed child leading to interrupted lactation and the cessation of the prohibition on cohabitation, with the likelihood that a woman will fall pregnant again quite soon after the loss of a child.

The causes of infant deaths following the breaking of postpartum sexual prohibitions are explained in different cultures in terms of a variety of beliefs. However, an association of some kind is frequently made between cohabitation, failure of the breast-feeding infant to thrive, short birth intervals and infant deaths. The Ghanaian work "Kwashiorkor" which means "the disease of the deposed baby when the next one is born" is now used universally to denote a syndrome of chronic protein and caloric deficiency in the two- to three-year-old weanling (Wray and Aguirre, 1966. See also Caldwell and Caldwell, 1977, pp. 198–201; Allen, 1967, p. 23; Molnos, 1972, pp. 12–16, 17–18). The Enga believe that it takes many acts of copulation to make a baby, and that gestation lasts for about eight months.[14] Therefore, although no exact sequential connection is made between a single act of intercourse and conception, pregnancy, lactational failure and deteriorating health in a still breast-feeding infant, a connection is certainly made between an act of coitus and the possible subsequent deterioration or even death of the infant. This is readily explained by the belief that the father's semen, which contains his war magic, mingles with the mother's milk within her body and kills the child.[15]

Western explanations of the risk of mortality associated with short birth intervals are, as we have seen, in terms of lessened intensity of maternal care, and/or of premature weaning, and the declining health status of the mother during and after pregnancy. However, the Enga explanation does provide a strong empirical rationale for prolonged birth intervals and is based on correct observation of mortality patterns; that is, if the rule of postpartum abstinence is broken, even once, the breast-feeding child and the next born may die. The death of the subsequent child is believed to be caused by the malevolent spirit of the dead elder sibling. Only when a child is about two and half years old, with full dentition, is its spirit believed strong enough to withstand total weaning, and the emotional upset of possible displacement by a new baby following on the resumption of parental cohabitation. At this age, its spirit is believed to be "strong" within its body and not likely to drift away due to dissatisfaction with this life, nor to be driven away by the malevolence of others, living or dead. It is at this point that Enga children are regarded as having a reasonable chance of survival—and so, given a name.[16]

Given all of the above mentioned factors, that is, the necessity of prolonged breast-feeding for the survival of infants and young children in the absence of nutritionally suitable and sterile weaning diets, the deleterious effect of pregnancy on lactation and the unreliability of lactational amenorrhoea in preventing conception, customary prolonged postpartum abstinence becomes the single most important means of ensuring the survival of infants and the maintenance of maternal health. Thus, the proscriptions which surround babies at the breast and their mothers, given the realities of Enga life, do enhance the survival chances of both.

The Age of Puberty in New Guinea Males

Although it may be argued that postpartum abstinence is based on objective observation of infant mortality patterns and that it contributes significantly to infant survival, I do not intend to look for a similar efficaciousness in the other practices to be discussed here, but simply to see whether or not their expressed aims are consistent with an objective observation of physiological processes. The first to be considered is puberty ritual and its relation to the age of puberty.

Throughout New Guinea, male puberty ritual is described by eth-

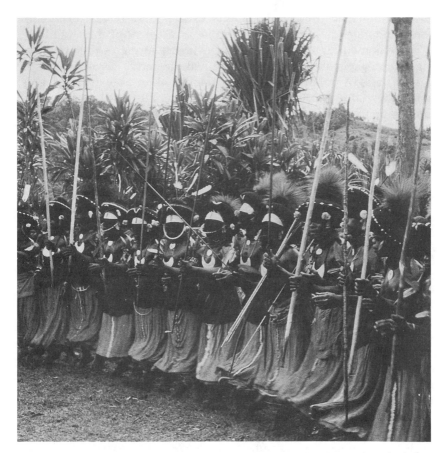

Fig. 1. In rituals expressing Enga anxiety over late age of puberty, these bachelors emerge from Sanggai ceremonies. They go through these ceremonies annually over a five year period.

nographers not only as a social *rite de passage*, but also as a means by which the participants believe that pubescence can be induced, its duration shortened and maturity more quickly attained. This could imply an indigenous dissatisfaction with the length of time taken to reach puberty. Indeed, ethnographers have found that pubescence, in boys at least, is regarded by many New Guinea societies as a prolonged and uncertain process. I am not suggesting that where such concerns are expressed by the people, puberty ritual will be important or will even exist. The presence of puberty ritual within a society cannot be explained so simply; but these ideas are always strongly expressed in puberty rites where they occur, and are usually a matter of importance even where they do not. Therefore, it seems reasonable to attempt some understanding of them and some assessment of their validity.

There is medical and demographic evidence available to support indigenous beliefs about attainment of male puberty. Throughout New Guinea, age of puberty is delayed, sometimes to an extreme degree, and pubescence is prolonged. Available data suggest that some New Guinea peoples attain maturity later than anywhere else in the world, but it must be remembered that such data are not available for many countries, especially large parts of Africa. If it were, perhaps the New Guineans would not seem unique in this respect. For example, Malcolm (1966) found that for the Bundi, where adequate records of the ages of subjects were available, the average age of *onset* of pubescence was 15.7 years for boys and 14.8 years for girls. The average age when sexual maturity was finally attained was 18.9 for boys and 18.8 for girls. These figures when compared with investigations in other countries show a relatively long delay in sexual development. Out of 109 Bundi girls, only one had menstruated by the age of seventeen. The development of the Bundi child of both sexes is slow, with a substantially longer period of pubescence (i.e. 4–6 years) than that found in European children (Malcolm, 1966, pp. 16–20).

Malcolm (1970) presents photographs of children and adolescents up to the age of 20, who look 3 to 5 years younger that their recorded ages. This is a reminder to the anthropologist of the subjective nature of relatively short term observations made in the field and the unreliability of age estimates based on the physical appearance of individuals.

Malcolm considers that the delayed development of the Bundi child is associated with nutritional factors (1970, p. 136). In this, he is supported by Tanner *et al.* (1966). Wark and Malcolm (1969, pp. 139 and 27) also associate slow development in the Lumi child with inadequate nutrition during childhood and adolescence. However, the Bundi present an extreme example of delayed development.

Sinnett (1977, p. 78) reports that growth in height and weight in Enga females is not completed until the age of 18 years, and in males not until 24 years. By contrast he quotes Tanner's figures for British children who reach adult stature by the age of 15 years in females and 17 years in males (Tanner *et al.*, 1966). Mission birth and baptismal records in the Laiagam area support this picture of late development in Enga children.

Sinnett implies that the Enga are comparable to the Chimbu in terms of relative dietary deficiencies and delayed development (Sinnett, 1977, p. 78; Malcolm, 1970, p. 296). He also suggests, in common with other researchers, that "the low protein content of the staple . . . [sweet potato] is the major factor imposing a serious limitation on the nutritional status of this population" (Sinnett, 1977, p. 70).

To give some idea of how this pattern of late puberty may be perceived by the members of a community, Malcolm points out that the Bundi "take nearly half their average life span in reaching maturity" (Malcolm, 1970, p. 2). The median age of attainment of puberty is about 18 years in boys. This implies that half of those reaching puberty will do so before this age, and the other half after. The latter individuals may be 19 to 20 years or more at puberty. This is a problem which particularly concerns the Enga, whose bachelor rites are held during the yearly dry season. In each clan, a relatively small group of about 500 individuals in which details of such events are easily known to the whole community, there are always a few boys who have been through the rites for four or five consecutive years and who are still "little boys", while their age-mates are fully mature.

Enga clan members believe that the relatively slow maturation of some of their bachelors is a sign that they are not adhering to traditional proscriptions with regard to the separation of the sexes. If a group cannot quickly bring their boys to maturity, they are considered by themselves, and by neighbouring groups, as neither producing enough warriors to protect themselves from hostile clans, nor enough husbands for the mature girls of those clans with whom they are allied by intermarriage.[17]

Researchers working in highland areas have often noted an indigenous uncertainty that all boys will reach manhood. This could be due to the lack of a definitive end-point in male maturation. In females, the onset of menstruation can be taken as an indication of adult status, and so problems of definition do not so clearly arise (see also Read, 1952, p. 15).

However, there is a further possible reason for this uncertainty. The Enga believe that if a boy did not go through the bachelor rites, he might never reach manhood in the physical sense, i.e. he could remain stunted and with an unbroken voice throughout life. It was also said that during the bachelor rites, boys risked growing breasts "like women" because of too close and frequent contact with the female *sanggai* plant (a type of bog iris) around which the rites were centred (Gray, 1972, p. 141). Malcolm mentions the incidence of enlarged male breasts or gyneacomastia in young adult Chimbu males (Malcolm, 1970, p. 296). Venkatachalam carried out a study of diet and nutrition in the Chimbu area in 1956–1957 and found that the prevalence of gyneacomastia was 10.3% among boys between 11 and 16 years of age, and occurred in 13.8% of adult males. It was more common among the younger adults of less than thirty years than in the older men. This condition has a complex etiology, but is believed to be associated with chronic protein and calorific undernutrition. It has also been reported in parts of India and Africa (Venkatachalam, 1962, p. 46).

Although gyneacomastia appeared to be rare in the Enga area during the late sixties, the people believed it to be common. Perhaps in the past it was, when pork, the main source of protein, was relatively scarce, and before the introduction of European high protein foodstuffs, such as tinned meat and fish, which are well utilized by the Enga today (Morren, 1977, p. 313).

By 1969–1970, the Yandapu Enga had been contacted by European patrols for about 15 years. Before this, endemic fighting and warfare, followed by propitiatary exchanges of large amounts of pork and other foodstuffs were said by the people to have depleted the pig population and to have caused recurrent famine. There is evidence of a similar pattern of recurrent famine following large exchanges of pork and sweet potato in the Chimbu area at a much later stage of European contact (Bailey, 1962a, p. 399). Furthermore, Enga gardens suffer from periodic frost damage, causing severe food shortages for the whole of the following season.

In 1969–1970 I knew of only one Enga male with gyneacomastia. He considered himself to be a woman and dressed as one, was married to a man (who had other wives) and did women's work. In the Laiagam area, even the existence of this single case of gyneacomastia, said by the people to have occurred in the four or five year period during which he was a participant in the bachelor rites, strongly influenced and supported symbolic representations within the rites, and served to confirm the uncertainties of the whole community with regard to male puberty.

A priori it seems unlikely that puberty ritual can influence processes of maturation; however, this does not deny that as with postpartum

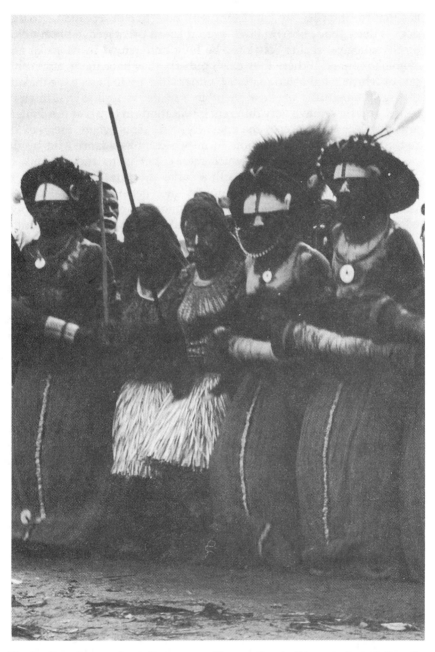

Fig. 2. Two dancers dressed as women. Transvestism in this context symbolizes the potency and warlike aggressiveness of men and women of the clan, against all other Enga clans.

abstinence, the rites are consistent with objective observation. Neither does it deny that puberty ritual, even if based on objective observation of physiological reality, can only be fully understood in its social and symbolic context. Where they exist, puberty rites have many aims, only one of which is to hasten maturity. Other aims are to hasten the making of, and the maturity of, "real men" in a social, as well as in a physical sense, and these have very different implications in terms of the content and the very existence of the rites. Even in areas where the rites do not exist, there is usually some form of sexual avoidance said by the people to be the means by which men either gain, and enhance or maintain, their masculinity in both a social and physical sense (Allen, 1967, p. 112). An understanding of why such beliefs are prevalent may perhaps be more easily reached if the ethnographer has a prior knowledge of those patterns of growth and maturation which constitute the norms in a given society, and upon which the expectations of its individual members may be founded. Anticipation of possible late maturity, based upon indigenous observation and taken in conjunction with the other biomedical factors described in this chapter may not, as such, explain the existence of puberty ritual, but are consistent with, and may be seen to provide, many of the ideas central to the symbolic content of the rites where they do exist, and of the social and ritual separation of the sexes in general.

Age of Puberty in New Guinea Females

In New Guinea, puberty in both sexes is delayed. However, perhaps because onset of menstruation is an end-point in female pubertal development, and occurs after other bodily changes, such as breast growth, have started, and because it dramatically marks a culmination in the whole process, age at menarche does not appear to be a source of anxiety.

Female maturity marked by menarche, even though it may be delayed, seldom fails to occur. At this point, a girl's fertility is taken for granted, and barrenness is dealt with in an *ad hoc* way if and when the problem arises later. Although there were indications of sub-fertility in the first year or so of marriage, there appeared to be little sterility among younger married women (Van de Kaa, 1971, p. 183, tables 6–15).

On the other hand, the traditional definition of a "real" man is one who is physically strong and personally aggressive both in warfare and in political and economic relationships with others; who is invulnerable to the malevolence of both the living and the dead and so invulnerable both to illness and to physical attack. These characteristics are not always achieved at puberty, even after undergoing the bachelor rites.

Male rites seem to concentrate on resolving not only physical uncertainties, but also those arising in dealings with both the ancestral and the spirit world, as well as with still living men. Large scale male puberty rites seem to constitute an attempt to resolve a complex of uncertainties both on a social and physical level, while female puberty rites at menarche are small, domestic affairs which celebrate a *fait accompli*. At this point, girls put on adult clothing and wear decorations and ornaments marking their father's wealth, and their own eligibility as future wives.

A sleek, fat body is regarded by the Enga as a most important physical asset in a young woman. A thin girl is considered unlikely to make a good marriage. From menarche onwards each girl undertakes a simple personal ritual which she carries out each day at dawn so that her body may grow fat, and her skin sleek and smooth.

The Enga recognize that illness and aging, especially in women, are always characterized by loss of weight (as will be shown in the following section). A fat woman is believed to live longer and her children more likely to survive. Yet there is no deliberate attempt to fatten marriageable girls.

However, during this time in their lives, girls are expected to attend all public gatherings and festivities, both large and small, held by their own and by neighbouring friendly clans. In this way they advertize their own attractions, as well as the success and prosperity of their clan. Because they frequently receive small gifts of pork and other foods during these occasions, which they usually consume on the spot, nubile girls probably do eat more than younger girls or older women. Furthermore, during the year or so before marriage girls certainly do less of the strenuous work generally expected of women.

It has been argued that there is a physiological mechanism whereby an increase to a critical ratio of fat to lean body weight must be reached before first menstruation can occur (Frisch and McArthur, 1974; Frisch, 1975). However, there is little clear evidence that such a critical ratio exists, although it has long been accepted that good nutrition and a higher body weight is associated with a relatively earlier onset of puberty in both sexes (Gray, 1977; Johnson *et al.*, 1975; Billewicz *et al.*, 1976; Trusswell, 1978).

In the Enga case, the higher nutritional intake and lower energy output of young women in the years before marriage does not occur until after menarche, and so cannot influence the age of its onset. The better diet of marriageable girls may reduce the numbers of adolescent anovulatory cycles but the available data suggests that the period of adolescent sub-fertility in New Guinea is, even so, relatively prolonged (Van de Kaa, 1971, p. 183, tables 6–15). However, the question must be left open until more detailed data are available.

The year or so during which girls enjoy relative ease and a probably better diet ends at marriage. Therefore, although women may be in a relatively good nutritional state for the first cycle of pregnancy and lactation, this is not true of subsequent pregnancies when, as we have seen, heavy nutritional demands are made. Therefore, a better diet and less strenuous life from menarche to marriage may shorten the period of post-pubertal infertility, but in the New Guinea situation, probably only marginally. After marriage, with the commencement of a heavy daily workload, and a return to the usual low protein diet, fertility would probably remain unaffected by the prior life style. There are data to suggest that there are high mortality rates among young girls throughout Melanesia (Van de Kaa, 1971, pp. 121, 145), therefore the years of relative ease and a better diet granted to Enga girls of marriageable age may enhance their survival chances, but there are no data from New Guinea which would enable one either to support or deny this conclusively.

In some areas of New Guinea and Melanesia, young girls are deliberately fattened during puberty ritual. However, such fattening is often carried out in association with a prior period of severe starvation or purging, frequently does not begin until after menarche has been reached and does not continue after marriage. Therefore, in most cases it could neither advance age of puberty nor increase fertility after marriage. Such feeding may shorten the period of adolescent sub-fertility, but where there is an initial period of starvation, even this must be in doubt.

The fattening of girls which occurs in some Melanesian societies has a parallel in the feeding of boys during male puberty ritual. Respectively, girls are fed "women's" foods (which are not always protein rich) and boys are fed "men's" foods. In Melanesia, it seems that such actions, for girls at least, because of the sequence of events, could have little physiological relevance to maturational processes or the establishment of fertility, and can therefore only be usefully analysed in conjunction with a study of the symbolism of male and female relationships. This symbolism is partly grounded in indigenous observations of physiological events, but the subject is too complex to be discussed fully here.

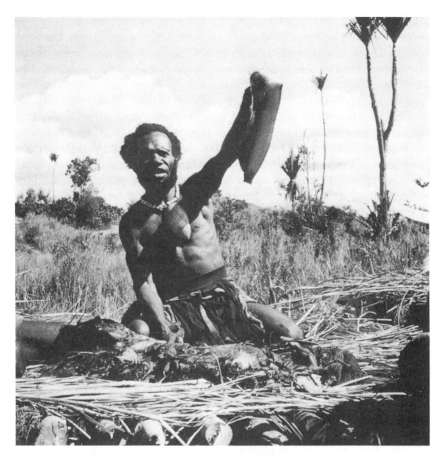

Fig. 3.   Distribution of pork at a public celebration.

The Premature Aging of Women in New Guinea

Although ritual behaviour may be based on valid perceptions of reality, the explanatory value of the biomedical data lies not in the ability to demonstrate the efficacy of ritual behaviour, nor of any one-to-one causal relationship, but simply in its ability to verify indigenous observations.

For instance, in so many areas of New Guinea, the social and ritual separation of the sexes is seen by the people as a means not only of allowing boys to grow into men, but also as a way of preventing men from becoming thin and weak early in life. The Enga believe that women experience rapid weight loss, muscle wasting and general debility from relatively early in life. Prohibitions surrounding menstruation, the blood of childbirth and the separation of the sexes in general were always explained by the Enga as the means by which men avoided these feminine afflictions (Meggitt, 1964; Gray, 1973, pp. 225–246). The medical and anthropological literature on New Guinea clearly supports this set of beliefs. In many areas of New Guinea, premature aging characterized by early weight loss is found in both sexes, but is more marked in women. Jelliffe and Maddocks (1964) have suggested that interrelated factors, such as under-nutrition and chronic infections of various kinds, in conjunction with the demands of menstruation, pregnancy, lactation and a heavy daily work load with a high energy expenditure, can lead to the premature aging of women.[18] They have referred to this as the "maternal depletion syndrome" (Jelliffe and Maddocks, 1964). Other researchers suggest that premature aging in women is more clearly associated with poor nutrition, that is, with nutritional intake not keeping pace with the requirements of an unusually strenuous life, with or without childbearing (Bailey, 1963; see also Vines, 1970; Wark and Malcolm, 1969; Malcolm, 1970; Sinnett, 1977). Bailey, in his study of the Chimbu, Baiyer river and Maprik areas, reported that weight for height showed a marked decline in women during their twenties. Men experienced a similar decline, but not until their thirties. He believed this to be the result of chronic protein deficiency throughout life. Also, skinfold thickness declined beyond 50 years in males, but throughout life in adult females, indicating a relative caloric sufficiency in males, but chronic caloric deficiency in females. Although Bailey found a distinct decline in the skinfold thickness of women with the occurrence of the first pregnancy/lactation cycle, he associated it with chronic undernutrition rather than with childbearing *per se*. The rationale for this conclusion was the observation that additional pregnancies after the first did not lead to further declines in skin folds, and all women showed a decline in height/weight ratios from the age of 25. However, it must be noted that the skinfold thicknesses reported by Bailey are so low that one would not expect any further significant declines since measurements below 3–4 mm represent the minimum thickness of skin in the absence of subcutaneous fat (personal communication, R. H. Gray). Therefore, although Bailey concluded that the main cause of physical deterioration and premature aging in women appeared to be strenuous and continuous activity, an inadequate diet, and chronic illness, the effects of pregnancy and lactation cannot be excluded (Bailey, 1963a, pp. 392–440; see also MacArthur, 1977, p. 111). This suggestion is further supported by Vines' work which shows that altered indices in height and weight in women from a relatively early age are found throughout New Guinea, including the Islands region, where nutrition is relatively good (Vines, 1970, pp. 273–274). However, differential distribution and consumption of food by the sexes may in part account for this.

Wark found that loss of height and weight in Lumi women began in the early twenties. Men, on the other hand, continued to gain weight until the mid-thirties and did not begin to lose it until they were in their forties (Wark and Malcolm, 1969, pp. 134–136). Wark also associated this steady decrease in female weight and height with chronic undernutrition and continuous and strenuous physical activity throughout life. Sinnett gives a broadly similar picture for the Enga and states that muscle loss, which is a major factor accounting for the age-related decrease in body weight experienced by the Enga, reflects their low protein intake (Sinnett, 1977, p. 80).[19] This fits well with the Enga emphasis on the progressive weakness and loss of weight which they experience and which, in men, they believe to result entirely from contact with women.

More recent data on the physiological relationship between lactating mothers and their suckling infants may be relevant to further understanding of the pattern of weight loss typical of women in New Guinea. Frequent feeding, or feeding on demand, is capable of maintaining high basal levels of the hormone prolactin (Delvoye *et al.*, 1977, p. 450). High levels of serum prolactin stimulate milk production and are associated with anovulation and long lasting postpartum amenorrhoea (ibid., p. 447). Lunn *et al.* have suggested that plasma prolactin concentrations during lactation also respond to changes in maternal diet. That is, when maternal diet is improved in under-nourished mothers, plasma prolactin concentrations are reduced at all stages of lactation (Lunn *et al.*, 1980). They also emphasize that demand feeding (at least between 10 and 16 times daily) is mainly confined to regions where there is a shortage of food. It would seem therefore that there might be a homeostatic compensatory mechanism, whereby even under conditions of chronic undernourishment, high levels of plasma prolactin enable the maintenance of successful lactation, with protein and calorie levels little below those of well fed western women (Whitehead *et al.*, 1978).

The metabolism and production of breast milk is extremely efficient. One study shows that in some areas the diet supplies only 150–200 kilocalories (which are units of 1000 calories) more than the daily basal and lactational calorie needs of lactating women. Where nutritional intake is inadequate to meet the energy and lactational requirements of the lactating mother there is evidence of a breakdown in maternal tissue to produce the fats and proteins necessary for adequate nutrition of the breast-feeding child (Jelliffe, 1976, p. 125). Only with frank starvation does milk volume drop and lactation gradually cease (Jelliffe and Jelliffe, 1977; Gopalan and Belavady, 1961). Even where milk volume is low due to severe maternal malnutrition, concentration of protein remains relatively high, so that overall protein output does not vary as greatly as one would expect between well nourished and poorly nourished women (Jelliffe and Jelliffe, 1977; Jelliffe, 1976, pp. 124–126; Belavady and Gopalan, 1960; Gopalan, 1958).

However, it must be pointed out that even with such lactational efficiency in the undernourished mother, her milk often falls short of satisfying the caloric demands of the growing child, since, although protein levels may remain high even where milk volume is low, the number of calories received by the child depends on the volume of milk digested daily (Jelliffe, 1976, p. 126; Jelliffe and Jelliffe, 1977; Whitehead et al., 1978, p. 179).[20] Furthermore, because of both great individual variation in the ability to increase and maintain milk volume, and in the time taken before ovulation is resumed, even in societies where demand feeding is practised and blood prolactin levels presumably high, postpartum abstinence may still be regarded as necessary in order to avoid early conception with resultant infant death.

As the other researchers in this field have done, Lunn et al. emphasize the effect heavy manual work and general physical exertion may have on the nutritional status of lactating mothers. Even when Gambian mothers had the same total mean dietary intake as the Cambridge (U.K.) mothers with whom they were compared in this study, "the relative adequacies of these intakes depended on considerable differences in patterns of heavy manual labour" (Lunn, 1980, p. 624; see also Gopalan, 1958, p. 91).

In conclusion, then, even where maternal nutrition appears to be good, that is, even where the diet appears to be as high in protein as it is in the Melanesian islands, or where disease rates and parasitic infestations such as malaria and hookworm appear to be low, nutritional intake may not be adequate to sustain the high energy requirements of a physically strenuous way of life, as well as the demands of pregnancies and lactation (Bailey, 1967a; Vines, 1970, pp. 273–274). It would seem then that loss of weight recorded in even relatively well nourished women in New Guinea may well be due to maternal nutritional depletion.[21]

The appearance of premature aging associated with rapid loss of weight and height is a real physical affliction of women in many areas of New Guinea, and stated to be so by the people themselves. The studies undertaken by Bailey, Vines, Malcolm and Wark are based on data covering two decades. Together with Sinnett's data, they provide a picture of the health status of a population not immediately observable to a research worker in the field for a relatively short time, but which may be fairly obvious to the people themselves over a generation. Certainly the Enga stressed their belief that women's reproductive powers made them age early, and be thin and weak and short-lived relative to men. This leads to two final points, concerning sex differentials in mortality and the reproductive life-span of women.

Sex Differences in Mortality Rates in New Guinea

When Enga men say that they avoid women and "women's things" in order to avoid an early death, their actions, although not efficacious, are consistent with a perception of relatively higher female mortality.

In New Guinea, diet is often sub-optional, no contraception or medical technology is available, chronic debilitating diseases are endemic, pregnancies are frequent, lactation long and maternal mortality high. In addition, the energy expenditure of women and the demands made upon their nutritional resources are throughout their lives consistently greater than those made upon men. Not surprisingly, therefore, where data are available, female mortality in the younger age groups is frequently higher than male mortality (see also Lewis, 1975, p. 105). Van de Kaa in his study of 1971, estimated that throughout Papua New Guinea, and contrary to the situation in the developed countries, the expectation of life of females is lower than that of males. There is an excess of female over male mortality, in infancy and in childhood, as well as during the childbearing years. Mortality rates among females begin to rise rapidly from the age of 10 years, whereas in males, rates do not begin to rise until their twenties, and then more slowly than they do in females (Van de Kaa, 1971, pp. 121, 145; see also "Nutrition and National Development", editorial comment in the Papua and New Guinea Medical Journal, vol. 12, No. 3, 1969, pp. 71–72).[22] Van de Kaa's findings are consistent with Vines' study of 1970.

Fertility in New Guinea

As a corollary to the arguments that New Guineans tend to mature late and grow old prematurely it would appear that under traditional circumstances, fertility would have been low and rates of natural increase nowhere near what they are today.

There is evidence that menarche is followed by a period of adolescent sub-fertility, which would explain the rarity of illegitimate births and the relatively low fertility of New Guinea women in the first years of marriage (Gray, 1977; Van de Kaa, 1971, p. 183, tables 6–15).[23]

There is also considerable evidence from New Guinea and other societies with poor nutrition that the menopause occurs at a relatively early age (Scragg, 1973; Gray, 1976, 1977; Wyon et al., 1966; Retel-Laurentin, 1977).

Given delayed menarche, the length of pregnancy, the long birth interval needed for maximum infant survival and early menopause, a woman's reproductive capacity is relatively limited. High infant and child mortality rates further decrease a woman's chances of having many children survive until maturity. Traditional investment in fertility ritual in the pre-contact era is consistent with biological pressures which restrict the individual's reproductive potential and the ability of the group to increase its numbers.

Conclusion

Most medical researchers and ethnographers who have worked in the New Guinea Highlands have been impressed by the strength and physical fitness of adults in their prime. However, to the peoples themselves, and the medical data support them in their view, this happy condition takes long to attain and lasts for a relatively short time, and many have not survived earlier critical life stages to enjoy it.

Furthermore, those who have survived, both in the traditional situation and even today, are vulnerable to illness or accident due to their way of life, the presence and the nature of endemic diseases, lack of the knowledge and amenities which make hygiene possible and the nutritional inadequacies of the traditional diet. Beyond this, the whole population, living as it does in marginal circumstances at high altitudes in the tropics and dependent on a non-storable staple, is vulnerable to sudden and total crop failure. This happened in 1972, when frost destroyed sweet potato mounds over wide areas of the highlands within a few days, leaving thousands with no food. A similar disaster had occurred previously in 1940–1941. Periodic famine has been described as a recurrent ecological situation for the Enga (Sinnett, 1977, p. 66; Binns, 1976; Brown and Powell, 1974).[24] The 1972 frost resulted in the emergence of the large scale propitiation rites which had fallen into disuse during the years of peace that coincided with Australian colonial administration (personal communication, Rev. H. Schaan).

Given these vicissitudes, the fit and active individuals, observed during a relatively limited period of field research, may well have valid expectations for a future rapid deterioration of their health status and life circumstances.

It has not been possible to discuss here the complicated question of whether types of political and economic organization (especially sexual biases in allocation of food and the sexual division of labour), or ecological factors, contribute most towards patterns of morbidity and aging, especially amongst women. These, and many other important issues must be considered elsewhere. My aim has been simply to demonstrate that observations of the health status and health practices of individuals and groups over a necessarily limited period of field research can be analysed in conjunction with data which places those events within a time frame allowing a reconstruction of the life cycle within a given society. Indigenous comprehension and expectations with regard to health and to patterns of critical life events can then be seen as plausible and the actions taken, whether efficacious or not, as rational, in the sense that they are consistent with the physical norms of that society.

Summary

The demographic picture presented for New Guinea, of high infant and child mortality rates, prolonged lactation and long birth intervals, delayed puberty, high mortality rates and premature aging, especially amongst women, is clearly consistent with indigenous statements.

(a) A prolonged postpartum prohibition on cohabitation does indeed facilitate the survival of infants, as it enables maternal care to be concentrated on each child, with lactation maintained for at least the first two years of life. The practice also safeguards maternal health and is appropriate to the ecological balance of food resources and maternal energy expenditure.

(b) Puberty is late and may not be achieved until half way through the individual's average life-span. New Guineans are amongst the world's latest maturers. The widespread belief that there is some uncertainty in boys achieving "real" manhood may be said to be based on indigenous observations of problems of maturation in areas where the traditional diet is lacking in important nutrients. Such observations and beliefs cannot be a sufficient explanation for the existence of puberty rites, but they do provide much of the thematic material in the rites where they occur. Since in this area aging is characterized by debility and loss of height and weight, and occurs much earlier in women, the separation of the sexes so that men may not become grey-haired, weak and thin or "skin-bone-nothing" (i.e. so that they will not become "like women") is comprehensible.

Large scale rites wherein the aim was to increase the fertility of gardens, pigs and women took place within a context of recurrent famine and low human fertility.[25]

Notes

(1) See also Vines (1970, p. 31).

(2) These and many other customary prescriptions and proscriptions are in general referred to by the word *Mana*. *Mana* in the Enga language means "traditional law" or "knowledge". Without *mana*, it is said that no man or woman can hope to gain success in any endeavour. To have *mana*, or to have knowledge of the law and to follow it, means, amongst other things, to obey all the Enga menstrual and sexual prohibitions. Men who attend the bachelor rites, and women who obey the rules of seclusion while menstruating and who correctly carry out the ritual return of menstrual blood to the ancestral life source, "have mana". They have not forgotten the law and are "real men" and "real women" (Glass, 1965, pp. 33, 41; Gray, 1973, pp. 101, 103). The word may have connections with the concept as it is found in other parts of Melanesia, but for the sake of brevity, this interesting question cannot be considered here.

(3) See also Caldwell and Caldwell (1977, pp. 198–199) for a similar explanation for postpartum prohibitions on intercourse in Nigeria and the reasons they give for not using the term "taboo". For example, in rural areas sexual relations are regarded as being tantamount to a physical assault on the baby (ibid., pp. 202–221).

(4) See Morren (1977, p. 313) and Buchbinder (1973) (cited by Morren) for evidence of recent population declines in certain isolated areas. During the late sixties, for example, the Hewa were believed by administration officers to be declining in numbers, due mainly to recurrent fighting and warfare (personal communication from D. Faithful, A.D.C. to the Lagaip sub-district until 1969).

There is evidence that the commencement of high rates of natural increase in the developing countries during this century is due to a fall in mortality rates at all ages but especially in infancy and childhood (Dyson, 1977, pp. 297–298). Rates of population increase in most developing countries rose dramatically after the second World War, with the use of antibiotics and sulphonamides.

The respiratory diseases to which New Guinea peoples seem to be so prone do not appear to have been introduced and have been the subject of prolonged medical debate. They contribute significantly to deaths in infants and in adults. The often fatal conditions similar to bronchitis so frequently seen in infants, and the chronic lung disease clinically resembling chronic bronchitis and emphysema experienced by adults, have been related to many factors, such as night-time temperatures, smoky house fires, malnutrition etc., and even to a particular kind of physiological adaptation to the utilization of carbon dioxide, said to be advantageous to the healthy, but not to the sick (Bayliss-Smith and Feacham, 1977, pp. 173–174; Sinnett and Whyte, 1973, pp. 267–268; Woolcock et al., 1970; Beral and Read, 1971). However, too little is known about the exact nature of these relationships to make definite statements on the etiology of this disease syndrome.

Even though medical technology can dramatically reduce the mortality rates associated with all of these factors, people today remain under-nourished and susceptible to disease and infection. Infant and childhood mortality rates are still high by western standards. These are the "diseases of poverty", which can only disappear in an area like New Guinea with major cultural, economic and technological change.

(5) In order to understand something of the pre-contact situation, it is necessary to exclude the introduced diseases, such as T.B., influenza, measles and whooping cough, which contribute to mortality rates today.

In the past, and still today, the two main causes of death in infancy and early childhood are diarrhoea and respiratory infections. The type of diarrhoea which so often killed young babies is referred to as "weanling diarrhoea" in the medical literature, and is not caused by pathogenic organisms so much as by the unsuitability of supplementary foods that are traditionally available (see the article by Biddulph and Pangkatana, 1971). Scragg, in his 1969 article on mortality declines in rural New Guinea, believed that the declines he observed were due mainly to the availability of medical technology—as there were few other changes at that time in the areas he studied. Sturt (1972, pp. 215–221) reported that infant mortality rates in the Sepik halved over a period of ten years, in an area with few changes other than the establishment of medical facilities and acceptance of them by the local population. He found no declines in the one to five years age groups (referred to by him as "toddlers") and put this down in part to the absence of a malaria control programme. Malaria accounted for 37% of deaths in this age group. Vines (1970) points out that urban dwellers and emigrants in New Guinea, although poor and often unemployed, have a better diet, better health status and lower mortality rates than do their contemporaries living in rural and still traditional mainland villages (Johnson, 1964; Davis, 1973; see also Van de Kaa, 1967).

The data provided by Vines (1970) and Sturt (1972) suggest that although medical technology can produce a dramatic fall in mortality rates, it may not change rates and patterns of morbidity where these are due to, for example, undernutrition caused by the nature of available foodstuffs, plentiful though these may, and to socio-economic factors. Therefore, high rates of natural increase in a population today cannot be taken to imply an overall improvement in the health status of most individuals in that population. Nor can this recent increase be used to support arguments for the adaptation to specific ecological conditions of New Guinea populations living under traditional circumstances in the past or even today.

(6) Sinnett, himself a doctor, also spent a large part of his time in the field providing much needed medical care. This may also account for the lower infant mortality rates which he recorded for the Murapin during his period of residence with them.

(7) The gastro-intestinal tract is sterile in fully breastfed babies. However, once even normal and necessary supplementary feeding begins, bacteriological cololization must occur. Even nonpathogenic bacteria can cause frequent and sometimes fatal diarrhoea (Biddulph and Pangkatana, 1971, pp. 7–13).

(8) Indeed, under traditional circumstances, there would have been little likelihood of a woman being able to do so due to relative undernutrition, and the high energy output required of women by traditional horticultural methods (see above, pp. 15–16 and 22–27).

(9) Contrary to the case in other areas, such as parts of Africa, the birth of twins, to the Enga, is associated with misfortune and affliction, and with the death and ill health of both women and children. It must be remembered that if a child dies or if its mother dies in childbirth (and there is a greater risk of this during multiple births) their spirits are, in this society, believed to be malevolent towards the living members of their group as are all spirits of the recently dead. Furthermore, the killing of one's child, or any member of one's lineage would normally mean immediate death at the hands of kinsmen.

(10) In theory, a child could also be fostered and adopted in exchange for a complicated series of payments to both its father's and to its dead mother's clans, but in practice this seldom seems to have been done.

(11) *Yama* refers to malevolent thoughts and to ill will in general. Those with *yama* may not know that they have it, although others may suspect them of it. So as not to seem to have it, and to prevent its powers being called into play if they do have it, people behave in socially acceptable ways so as not to be branded as one with *yama*. When a person dies, a post-mortem operation is always carried out to decide the cause of death and from whom compensation must be demanded. It is at this time that *yama*, or "black blood", may be discovered in the body of the deceased and the question finally settled (see also Evans-Pritchard, 1937, pp. 9, 21–23).

(12) Ooman in 1956 said, of New Guinea children, that he believed it was the "toddler", not the suckling, who was at risk. The WHO report of 1977 (Dyson, 1977, p. 282) suggests that indeed, "child mortality", i.e. up to 5 years, may be as high, and sometimes higher than, mortality in infancy, with perhaps the highest mortality during the second year of life. In New Guinea, and in many other parts of the Third World, the two-year-old has often been recently weaned. Those at risk are the ones who have experienced the cycle already described of recurrent infections leading to malnutrition and further derangement of the immune response. Kwashiorkor and marasmus are typical afflictions of the weanling.

(13) Intensity of suckling varies depending upon whether an infant is fully or partially breast-fed. Although a child ideally will be breast-fed for more than two years, it will also require supplementary foods from approximately six months onwards. Although the amount of milk consumed daily will still be large, as an older child takes more at a single feed, intensity of suckling will be reduced (see Rowland *et al.*, 1978, pp. 136–137; this study gives some indication of frequency of feeding and amounts of milk consumed daily).

(14) Enga mothers believed that a pregnancy lasting longer than this could lead to a large foetus and an obstructed labour. Therefore, during the last weeks of pregnancy, women often work harder in their gardens and indulge in other strenuous activities in order to induce labour.

(15) Therefore, as Enga mothers frequently said, "If we had European baby foods, we would have no need for postpartum abstinence,

as we would not have to breast-feed our babies". The problem could not, of course, be solved so simply, as non-sterile baby foods or cows' milk fed to infants under unhygienic conditions would still be dangerous to the child (Muller, 1974; Gray, 1975), but the point made is in principle correct.

(16) Not naming a child until it is two years or more is based on an awareness of high infant and early childhood mortality rates. The name of a deceased person may not be mentioned or given to another for many years, for fear of calling up the malevolent spirit. It is said, therefore, that if all babies of under two were named, a proliferation of personal names of unmanageable proportions would result. The practice of not naming infants and very young children is sometimes believed by the outsider to be an indication of a fatalistic acceptance of death. However, the dramatic severity of mourning practices—the amputation of fingers etc., even for young babies—seemed to me to be more expressive of grief, despair and fear of the dead, even if not of death itself.

(17) See Gray (1973, pp. 19–23) for a discussion of Yandapu Enga marriage choices. Here, marriage with traditionally friendly groups, and not with enemies, was always favoured.

(18) For instance, in the Highlands, anaemia in women is very common (WHO, 1968), and is probably due to the low iron content of the diet; the loss of iron associated with menstruation together with diseases such as malaria and hookworm, and in married women, with pregnancy and lactation (Drover and Maddocks, 1975; Stanhope, 1975). Even in the U.K., where a high protein diet is available, anaemia in pregnancy is common enough for iron and folic acid to be prescribed as a routine part of antenatal care.

(19) Sinnett reports that Enga body weight reaches a maximum between the ages of 20 and 29 years. Therefore, both sexes show a progressive decline in body weight with advancing age, men losing 23.3% of their body weight between the third and seventh decades of life, while women experience a weight reduction of 25% during the same period. Because of his different research aims, Sinnett does not give details of changing rates with age for each sex. Nor does he say how he calculated the ages of individuals within his study. There is recent demographic evidence to suggest that in many such societies in the underdeveloped world, the proportions of the population surviving to the seventh decade of life would be very small (Gray, 1977). Becroft et al. in a study of the Kyaka Enga of the Baiyer River found that in their calculated age distribution of the population, they had a relative deficiency of persons

aged 20 to 34, and a relatively high number of old people. They considered that this suggested an over-estimation of numbers of middle-aged and elderly subjects at the expense of young adult age groups (Becroft *et al.*, 1969, p. 51). This may be indicative of early aging, where sudden declines in weight from the mid-twenties onwards would bias subjective age estimation. Despite these drawbacks, Sinnett's description of Enga nutritional status is valuable in its detail and is similar in its general emphasis to those given for the Chimbu, Baiyer River, Mapric and Lumi areas (Sinnett, 1977, p. 80).

(20) It is important to note that although breast milk makes a valuable contribution to the nutritional requirements of a child over prolonged periods, requirements for infant growth may not be fully met, for although the quality of her milk is high, the undernourished mother has a lower yield.

In Gambia for instance, "breast milk intake did not increase with age to meet the raised nutritional needs of the growing child. There was little change in mean milk intake over the first 3 months of lactation; thereafter it fell progressively. Only with the first child did breast milk intake rise beyond 3 months to meet the increasing needs of the growing child" (Whitehead *et al.*, 1978, p. 179). "In spite of an adequate suckling stimulus and opportunities for feeding, the mothers in this study were unable to respond by increasing milk yield" (ibid, p. 180).

(21) The recommended dietary intake by the U.S. National Academy of Sciences takes into account the maintenance of a reserve of maternal subcutaneous fat which is believed to contribute at least 300 kilocalories daily to lactation output for about three to four months, and which is also believed to supply vitamin and essential fatty acids, which are often low in the breast milk of undernourished mothers (Jelliffe, 1976, p. 120; National Academy of Sciences, 1974).

Jelliffe points out that loss of weight during lactation is common. Poorly nourished women may lose up to 7 kg in weight after one year of lactation, and nutritional oedema has been reported in some women. Indeed, the weight of poorly nourished women may not change during lactation, and it has been suggested that tissue loss is hidden by increases in the amount of body water, in other words, by nutritional oedema, in very poorly nourished women (Jelliffe, 1976, p. 128).

(22) Within the 35 to 39 years age group in New Guinea, the sex differences in mortality patterns begins to change, and by this

stage in the life cycle, the death rates in both sexes are comparable. By the age of 40 years, male mortality begins to exceed female mortality, as it does in the developed countries, even though mortality rates are higher for women in the younger age groups (Van de Kaa, 1971, p. 118, table 5). In other words, female life expectancy when calculated from any point in the first three decades of life, is lower than that for males; but for those women who survive these decades, life expectancy from about the age of forty years is, as we find in the west, as high, or higher than for men.

Maternal mortality rates for any underdeveloped country are difficult to estimate (Tietz, 1977, pp. 312–317). However, Babona *et al.* suggest that the rates for New Guinea as a whole may be somewhere between six and ten per 1000 births (Babona *et al.*, 1974, p. 331).

(23) Frisch has demonstrated a close association with body weight and the onset of menarche. She has gone further and suggested that body weight may be a critical factor leading to the onset of menarche (Frisch and McArthur, 1974; Frisch, 1975). Although the former association has been accepted by most researchers, the latter hypothesis has been questioned by other authors (Gray, 1977, pp. 221, 227; Johnson *et al.*, 1975; Billewicz *et al.*, 1976).

(24) The median estimates were calculated on augmented data by J. Barrett and R. H. Gray. An association has also been suggested between earlier menopause, and low body weight and height (Gray, 1977, p. 227).

(25) Periodic migration due to famine and to warfare, and the effect this may have had on the social structure of various Highlands societies, as well as upon the dissemination of customs and beliefs, is a further point of interest which has not been discussed in this chapter.

References

Addo, N. O. and Goody, J. (1974). *Siblings in Ghana*. Department of Social Anthropology, Cambridge, and the Institute of Social Economic Research, Legon, Ghana.

Allen, M. R. (1967). *Male Cults and Secret Initiations in Melanesia*. Melbourne: Melbourne University Press.

Babona, G., Bird, G. D. and Johnson, D. G. (1974). "Maternal Mortality in Papua New Guinea". *Papua New Guinea Medical Journal* **17**, 331–334.

Bailey, K. V. (1963). "Nutritional Status of East New Guinea Populations". *Tropical and Geographical Medicine* **15**, 389–402.

Bayliss-Smith, T. P. and Feacham, R. G. (1977). "Subsistence and Survival". In *Rural Ecology in the Pacific*. London: Academic Press.

Becroft, T. C., Stanhope, J. and Burchett, P. M. (1969). "Mortality and Population Trends Among the Kyaka Enga, Baiyer Valley". *Papua New Guinea Medical Journal* **12**, 48–55.

Belavady, B. and Gopalan, C. (1960). "Effect of Dietary Supplementation on the Composition of Breast Milk". *Indian Journal of Medical Research* **48**, 518–222.

Beral, V. and Read, D. J. C. (1971). "Insensitivity of the Respiratory Centre to Carbon Dioxide in the Enga People of New Guinea". *Lancet* **2**, 1290.

Biddulph, J. and Pangkatana, P. (1971). "Weanling Diarrhoea". *Papua New Guinea Medical Journal* **14**, 7–13.

Biersteker, K. (1961). "Infant Mortality in Netherlands Papua New Guinea". *Papua New Guinea Medical Journal* **5**, 11.

Billewiez, W. Z., Fellowes, H. M. and Hythen, C. A. (1976). "Comments on the Critical Metabolic Mass and the Age of Menarche". *Annals of Human Biology* **3**, 51–59.

Binns, C. W. (1976). "Famine and the Enga". *Papua New Guinea Medical Journal* **19**, 231–235.

Brown, M. and Powell, J. M. (1974). "Frost and Drought in the Highlands of New Guinea". *Journal of Tropical Geography* **38**, 1.

Buchbinder, G. (1973). Maring microadaptation: a study of demographic nutritional, genetic and phenotypic variation in a highland New Guinea population. Ph.D. Dissertation in Anthropology, Columbia University, New York.

Caldwell, J. C. and Caldwell, P. (1977). "The Role of Sexual Abstinence in Determining Fertility: A Study of the Yoruba in Nigeria". *Population Studies* **31**, 2.

Cantrelle, P. and Leridon, A. (1971). "Breast Feeding, Mortality in Childhood and Fertility in a Rural Zone of Senegal". *Population Studies* **25**, 505–533.

Crane, G. G. and Kelly, A. (1972). "The Effect of Malaria Control on Haematological Parameters in the Kaiapit Sub-District". *Papua New Guinea Medical Journal* **15**, 38–44.

Davis, K. (1973). "Cities and Mortality". *IUSSP Population Conference, Liege*, **3**, 259.

Delvoye, P., Demaegd, M., Delogne-Desnoeck, J. and Robyn, C. (1977). "The Influence of the Frequency of Nursing and of Previous Lactation on Serum Prolactin in Lactating Mothers". *Journal of Biosocial Science* **9**, 447–451.

Drover, K. and Maddocks, I. (1975). "Iron Content of Native Foods". *Papua New Guinea Medical Journal* **18**, 15–17.

Dyson, T. (1977). "Levels, Trends, Differentials and Causes of Child Mortality—A Survey". *WHO Statistics Report* **30**, 282–311.

Editorial (1955–1956). "Our Duties". *Papua New Guinea Medical Journal* **1**, 33.

Editorial (1969). "Nutrition and National Development". *Papua New Guinea Medical Journal* **12**, 71–72.

Editorial (1975–1976). "Ascaris Infection and Malnutrition in Tropical Children". *Papua New Guinea Medical Journal* **1**, 36.

Evans-Pritchard, E. E. (1937). *Witchcraft, Oracles and Magic Among The Azando*. Oxford: Clarendon Press.

Frisch, R. E. (1975). "Demographic Implications of the Biological Determinants of Female Fecundity". *Social Biology* **22**, 17–22.

Frisch, R. E. and McArthur, J. W. (1974). "Menstrual Cycles: Fatness as a Determinant of Minimum Weight for Height Necessary for their Maintenance or Onset". *Science* **185**, 949–951.

Frood, J. D. L., Whitehead, R. G. and Coward, W. A. (1971). "Relationship Between Pattern of Infection and Development of Hypoalbuminaemia and Hypo-B-Lipoproteinaemia in Rural Ugandan Children". *Lancet* **11**, 1047–1049.

Glass, R. M. (1965). "The Huli of the Southern Highlands". In *Gods, Ghosts and Men in Melanesia* (P. Laurence and M. J. Meggitt, eds). Melbourne: Oxford University Press.

Gopalan, C. (1958). "Studies in Lactation in Poor Indian Communities". *Journal of Tropical Paediatrics* **4**, 87–92.

Gopalan, C. and Belavady, B. (1961). "Nutrition and Lactation". *Federation Proceedings (Suppl. 4)* **20**, 177–183.

Gopalan, C. and Nadamuni Naidu, A. (1972). "Nutrition and Fertility". *Lancet* **11**, 1077–1079.

Gordon, J. E., Chitkara, I. D. and Wyon, J. B. (1962). "Weanling Diarrhoea". *American Journal of Medical Science* **245**, 345–377.

Gray, B. M. (1973). The logic of Yandapu Enga puberty rites and the separation of the sexes: responses to ecological and biological pressures in New Guinea. Thesis presented for the M.A. degree in the Department of Social Anthropology, University of Sydney, May 1973.

Gray, R. H. (1974). "Re-assessment of the Contribution of Malaria Control, Health Services, Nutrition and Economic Development". *Population Studies* **28**, 205–229.

Gray, R. H. (1975). "Breast-Feeding and Maternal and Child Health". *IPPF Medical Bulletin* **9**, 1–3.

Gray, R. H. (1976). "The Menopause, Epidemiological and Demographic Considerations", pp. 25–40. Lancaster: MTP. In *The Menopause* (R. Beard, ed.).

Gray, R. H. (1977). Biological factors other than nutrition and lactation which may influence natural fertility: a review. In *Natural Fertility* (H. Leridon and J. Menken, eds), pp. 217–250. Liege: IUSSP.

Hogbin, H. I. (1943). "A New Guinea Infancy". *Oceania* **13**, 285–309.

Jain, A. K., Hermalin, A. J. and Sun, T. H. (1977). Lactation and natural fertility. IUSSP seminar on "Natural Fertility", INED, Paris, pp. 1–34.

Jelliffe, D. B. and Maddocks, J. (1964). "Notes on Ecological Malnutrition in the New Guinea Highlands". *Clinical Paediatrics* **3**, 432–438.

Jelliffe, E. F. P. (1976). Maternal nutrition and lactation. In *Breastfeeding and the Mother*, pp. 119–143. Ciba Foundation Symposium 45, (New Series), New York.

Jelliffe, D. B. and Jelliffe, E. F. P. (1977). *Human Milk in the Modern World*. Oxford: Oxford University Press.

Johnson, G. Z. (1964). "Health Conditions in Rural and Urban Areas of Developing Countries". *Population Studies* **17**, 293.

Johnston, F. E., Roche, A. R., Schell, L. M. and Wettenhal, H. N. B. (1975). "Critical Weight of Menarche: Critique of a Hypothesis". *American Jounal of Diseases of Childhood* **129**, 19–23.

Lewis, G. (1975). *Knowledge of Illness in a Sepik Society: A Study of the Gnau, New Guinea*. LSE Monographs on Social Anthropology, No. 52. London: Athlone Press.

Lunn, P. C., Austin, S., Prentice, A. M. and Whitehead, R. G. (1980). "Influence of Maternal Diet on Plasma-prolactin Levels during Lactation". *Lancet*, March 22, 623–625.

MacArthur, M. (1977). "Nutritional Research in Melanesia: a Second Look at the Tsembaga". In *Subsistence and Survival Rural Ecology in the Pacific* (T. P. Bayliss-Smith and R. G. Feacham, eds), pp. 91–128. London: Academic Press.

Malcolm, L. A. (1966). "The Age of Puberty in the Bundi People". *Papua New Guinea Medical Journal* **9**, 16–20.

Malcolm, L. A. (1969). "Child Mortality and Disease Patterns—Recent Changes in the Bundi Area". *Papua New Guinea Medical Journal* **12**, 13–18.

Malcolm, L. A. (1970). *Growth and Development in New Guinea: A Study of the Bundi People of the Madang District, Madang*. New Guinea Institute of Human Biology. Monograph Series, No. 1.

Meggitt, M. J. (1964). "Male-Female Relationships in the Highlands of Australian New Guinea". *American Anthropologist*, Special Publication, **66**, 204–224.

Meggitt, M. J. (1965). "The Mae Enga of the Western Highlands". In *Gods, Ghosts and Men in Melanesia* (P. Lawrence and M. J. Meggitt, eds), pp. 129–130. Melbourne: Oxford University Press.

Molnos, A. (1972). *Cultural Source Materials for Population Planning in East Africa*. Nairobi: East African Publishing House.

Morley, D. (1973). In *Paediatric Priorities in the Developing World*, pp. 100–123. London: Butterworths.

Morren, George E. B. (1977). "From Hunting to Herding: Pigs and the Control of Energy in Montane New Guinea". In *Subsistence and Survival: Rural Ecology in the Pacific* (T. P. Bayliss-Smith and R. G. Feacham, eds), pp. 273–316. London: Academic Press.

Morrison, S. L., Heady, J. A. and Morris, J. N. (1959). "Mortality in the Post-Neonatal Period". *Archives of Diseases in Childhood* **34**, 101–114.

Muller, M. (1974). *The Baby Killer*. London: War On Want.

National Academy of Sciences (1974). *Recommended Dietary Allowances*, 8th Edition, Washington, D.C.

Nichol, B. M. (1971). "Protein and Calorie Concentration". *Nutrition Reviews* **29**, 83–88.

Nutrition and National Development (1969). Editorial. *Papua New Guinea Medical Journal* **12**, 71–72.

Nutrition Reviews (1972). *Cellular Immunity and Malnutrition* **30**, 253.

Omran, A. R. and Standley, C. C. (1976). *Family Formation Patterns and Health*. Geneva: World Health Organization.

Oomen, H. A. P. C. (1956). "Assessment and Prevention of Child Malnutrition". *Papua New Guinea Medical Journal* **2**, 1–20.

Oomen, H. A. P. C. and Cordon, M. W. (1970). *Metabolic Studies in New Guineans: Nitrogen Metabolism in Sweet Potato Eaters*. South Pacific Commission Technical Paper, No. 163.

Posala, H. F. (1969). "Customs and Beliefs in Relation to Health and Disease in the Kainantu Sub-district". *Papua New Guinea Medical Journal* **12**, 91–95.

Puffer, R. R. and Serrano, L. V. (1973). In *Patterns of Mortality in Childhood*. PAHO Report on the Inter-American Investigation of Mortality in Childhood, pp. 1–38.

Read, K. E. (1952). "Nama Cult of the Central Highlands, New Guinea". *Oceania* **23**, 1–25.

Retel-Laurentin, A. (1977). In *Quelques éléments de la fecondité naturelle dans deux population africaines à faible fecondité*. Distributed at the Seminar on Natural Fertility, INED/IUSSP, Paris, pp. 1–20.

Rowland, M. G. M., Barrell, R. A. E. and Whitehead, R. G. (1978). "The Weanling's Dilemma: Bacterial Contamination in Traditional Gambian Weaning Foods". *Lancet*, Jan. 21, 136–138.

Schonland, M. (1973). "Depression of Immunity in Protein-Calorie Malnutrition: A Post-Mortem Study". *Journal of Tropical Paediatrics and Environmental Child Health* **3**, 217–224.

Scragg, R. F. R. (1957). *Depopulation in New Ireland (Territory of Papua New Guinea)*. TPNG Health Department, Monograph No. 15.

Scragg, R. F. R. (1969). "Mortality Changes in Rural New Guinea". *Papua New Guinea Medical Journal* **12**, 73–90.

Scragg, R. F. R. (1973). In *Menopause and Reproductive Span in Rural Nugini*. Presented at the Annual Symposium of the Papua New Guinea Medical Society, p. 126, Port Moresby.

Scrimshaw, N. S., Taylor, L. E. and Gordon, J. E. (1968). In *Interactions of Nutrition and Infection*. WHO Monograph Series, No. 57, p. 329. Geneva: World Health Organization.

Sinnett, P. F. (1977). "Nutrition Adaptation among the Enga". In *Subsistence and Survival: Rural Ecology in the Pacific* (T. P. Bayliss-Smith and Richard G. Feachman, eds). Academic Press: London.

Sinnett, P. F. and Whyte, H. M. (1973). "Epidemiological Studies of a Highland Population of New Guinea: Environment, Culture and Health Status". *Human Ecology Journal* No., 245–277.

Srikantia, S. G., Siva Prasad, J., Braskaram, C. and Krishnamach-ari, K.A.V.R. (1976). "Anaemia and Immune Response". *Lancet* **1**, 1307.

Stanhope, J. M. (1975). "Anaemia in the Lower Rama Area". *Papua New Guinea Medical Journal* **18**, 8–11.

Stoeckel, J. and Chowdhury, A.K.M.A. (1972). "Neo-natal and Post-neo-natal Mortality in a Rural Area of Bangladesh". *Population Studies* **26**, 113–120.

Sturt, J. (1972). "Infant and Toddler Mortality in the Sepik". *Papua New Guinea Medical Journal* **15**, 215–221.

Tanner, J. M., Whitehouse, R. H. and Takaishi, M. (1966). "Standards from Birth to Maturity for Height, Weight, Velocity and Weight Velocity for British Children". *Archives of Diseases in Childhood* **41**, 454–613.

Tietz, C. (1977). *Maternal Mortality Excluding Abortion Mortality*. World Health Statistics Report, Vol. 30, No. 4. Geneva: World Health Organization.

Trusswell, J. (1978). "Menarche and Fatness: Re-examination of the Critical Body Composition Hypothesis". *Science* **200**, 1506–1509.

Tyson, J. E., Freedman, R. S., Perez, A., Zacur, H. A. and Zarnatur, J. (1976). "Significance of the Secretion of Human Prolactin and Gonadotrophin for Pueperal Lactational Infertility". In *Breast-feeding and the Mother*, pp. 49–71. CIBA Foundation Symposium 45. Elsevier, Exerpta Medica.

Vallin, J. (1976). In *World Trends in Infant Mortality Since 1950*, pp. 646–673. WHO Statistics Report, Vol. II.

Van de Kaa, D. J. (1967). "Medical Work and Changes in Infant Mortality in Western New Guinea". *Papua New Guinea Medical Journal* **10**, 89.

Van de Kaa, D. J. (1971). The demography of Papua and New Guinea's indigenous population. Ph.D. Thesis, ANU, Canberra.

Van Ginneken, J. K. (1974). "Prolonged Breast-feeding as a Birth Spacing Method". *Studies in Family Planning* **5**, 201–206.

Van Zijl, W. J. (1966). "Studies of Diarrhoeal Diseases in Seven Countries". *World Health Organization Bulletin* **35**, 249–261.

Venkatachalam, P. S. (1962). *A Study of the Diet, Nutrition and Health of the People of the Chimbu Area (New Guinea Highlands).* Department of Public Health, Monograph, No. 4, Territory of Papua New Guinea.

Vines, A. P. (1970). *An Epidemiological Sample Survey of the Highlands, Mainland and Island Regions of the Territory of Papua New Guinea.* Territory of Papua New Guinea Health Department, Port Moresby.

Wark, L. and Malcolm, L. A. (1969). "Growth and Development of the Lumi Child in the Sepik District of New Guinea". *Medical Journal of Australia* **2**, 129–136.

Whitehead, R. G., Hutton, M., Müller, E., Rowland, M. G. M., Prentice, A. M. and Paul, A. (1978). "Factors Influencing Lactation Performance in Rural Gambian Mothers". *Lancet,* July 22, 178–181.

WHO (1968). *Scientific Group on Nutritional Anaemias.* Geneva: WHO Technical Report Series 405.

WHO (1973). *Energy and Protein Requirements.* Report of a Joint FAO/WHO Ad Hoc Expert Committee (1973). WHO Technical Report Series 522.

Wolfers, D. and Scrimshaw, S. (1975). "Child Survival and Intervals Between Pregnancies in Guayaquil, Ecuador". *Population Studies* **29**, 479–495.

Woolcock, A. J., Blackburn, C. R., Freeman, M. H., Zylstra, W. and Spring, S. R. (1970). "Studies of Chronic (Non-tuberculous) Lung Disease in New Guinea Populations. The Nature of the Disease". *American Review of Respiratory Diseases* **102**, 575–590.

Wray, J. D. (1971). "Population Pressure on Families: Family Size and Child Spacing". *Reports on Population Studies in Family Planning* **9**, 403–460.

Wray, J. D. and Aguirre, A. (1969). "Protein-calorie Malnutrition in Candelaria, Colombia: 1, Prevalence, Social and Demographic Causal Factors". *Journal of Tropical Pediatrics* **15**, 76–98.

Wyon, J. B. and Gordon, J. E. (1962). "A Long-term Prospective-type Field Study of Population Dynamics in the Punjab, India". In *Research in Family Planning* (C. V. Kiser, ed.), pp. 17–32. Princeton: Princeton University Press.

Wyon, J. B., Finner, S. L. and Gordon, J. E. (1966). "Differential Age at Menopause in Rural Punjab, India". *Population Index* **32**, 328.

4. Health, Fertility and Birth in Moyamba District, Sierra Leone

C. P. MacCormack

Introduction: Practice and Innovation

A women's organization concerned with maintaining health and fertility has functioned in coastal southern Sierra Leone at least since the 1600s when it was described by the Dutch geographer Dapper (Fyfe, 1964, pp. 35–40). This women's sodality, the Sande society, organized in virtually every village in Sierra Leone today (see MacCormack, 1979). The senior officials of each local chapter, and a few younger women who display special adeptness, deliver maternal and child care and treat certain categories of illness. Sande's function is complemented by that of the men's sodality, Poro, which for centuries has been concerned with such public health policies as clean wells and conservation of food resources. This paper will concentrate upon the Sande society, but with the clear proviso that gender complementarity is central to Mende and Sherbro thought (MacCormack, 1981).

According to a recent survey, no one in Sierra Leone lives more than three miles from a Sande practitioner (Minette, 1980). This organization is an excellent indigenous social structure upon which to "invest" additional training in Western medical knowledge and basic medical supplies. The personnel are "of" the villages and will not go away after training. They are supported by an ancient, accepted, non-exploitive fee-for-service system. The practitioners have "traditional legitimacy" (in a Weberian sense) and can act with authority. Because the practi-

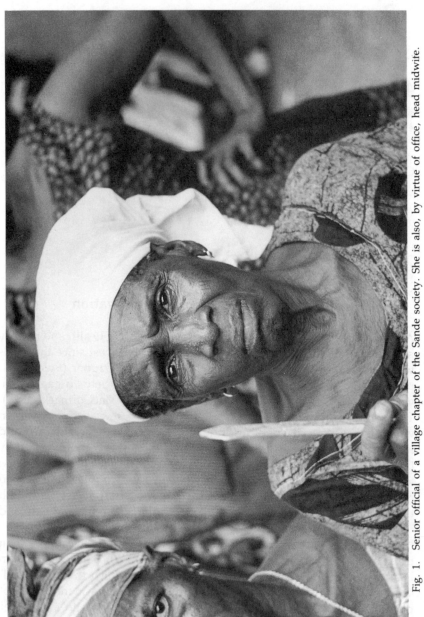

Fig. 1. Senior official of a village chapter of the Sande society. She is also, by virtue of office, head midwife.

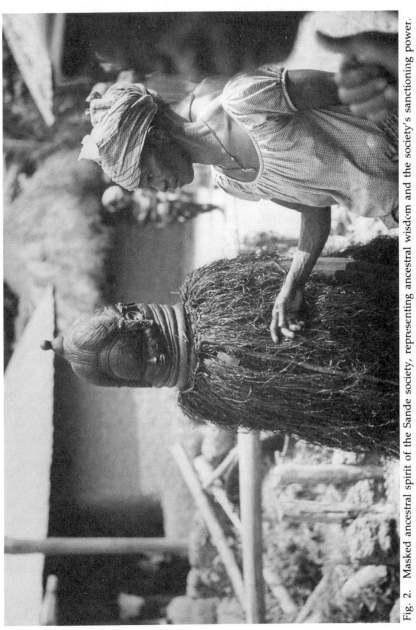

Fig. 2. Masked ancestral spirit of the Sande society, representing ancestral wisdom and the society's sanctioning power.

tioners *achieve* their roles by acquiring adeptness in practice of the healing arts, rather than having them *ascribed* by heredity, they are eager to learn new therapies and new preventive techniques in order to enhance their reputation and social standing in their local area.

Although these practitioners are eager to integrate their knowledge with what they judge to be useful in Western cosmopolitan medicine, Western trained doctors have been for the most part either indifferent or hostile to practitioners in the Sande society. If acknowledged at all, they are called "traditional birth attendants", connoting women who stand about rather passively while birth as a "natural" process, or a medical process for which they only marginally qualify to take a role, takes its course. But as this chapter seeks to demonstrate, birth is also a cultural and a social process. Sande midwives are towering figures in a village, communicating confidence and authority in both speech and body language (Kargbo, 1975). Some are town chiefs, section chiefs, and all but one of the 12 women paramount chiefs in Sierra Leone are high ranking Sande women (MacCormack, 1972). They enhance their reputation with successful health care. Indeed, as political figures they are morally obliged to do all they can to protect and maintain the health and fertility of their people.

Because Sande officials' status is achieved rather than ascribed, they have often responded quickly to medical innovations. In the 1940s, Milton Margai, a Mende physician who became Sierra Leone's first post-independence prime minister, was well aware that Sande women were keen to learn more effective medical practices, providing their autonomy was not jeopardized nor their secret corporate knowledge revealed. Dr. Margai worked through prominent paramount chiefs, especially women paramount chiefs in Sande, to introduce additional information about anatomy and physiology, venereal diseases, sanitation, first aid and other knowledge about basic hygiene (Margai, 1948).

Since then, Sande midwives have volunteered readily for the few places in training programmes for "traditional birth attendants", and recently have cooperated enthusiastically with culturally appropriate health education programmes. They have taken songs, tape-recorded songs and domestic drama, and illustrated "short talks" to their villages to teach others about such things as improved weaning foods (Minette, 1980).

Any truly appropriate primary health care system in Sierra Leone cannot be narrowly based upon the Western "engineering" approach to medicine where chemicals are prescribed as quickly and efficiently as possible for faulty organs. Rather, an appropriate system will have to recognize disease in whole persons embedded within social and moral contexts. This chapter, focused upon maternal and child health, is an attempt to explicate some of that context, and meld it together with Western medical discourse.

The Setting

Moyamba District is inhabited primarily by people of Mende, and Sherbro, language and culture; Mende in the interior and Sherbro in the coastal area. The economy is based upon shifting cultivation of rice and cassava with some shallow-water fishing. Increasingly people are turning from land extensive cultivation to labour intensive swamp rice cultivation (MacCormack, 1978). The population density today is just under 100 people per square mile and was probably much lower in the nineteenth century. In the coastal area particularly, land is swampy with malaria, schistosomiasis and other tropical diseases debilitating the population. In 1970, women in rural villages, aged 40 to 49, had given birth on average to 8.5 children with 3.9 children surviving (Dow, 1972). The health and fertility of people and the land are constant preoccupations, expressed most notably in beliefs about laws of behaviour handed down from ancestors and ancestresses in a system of descent groups[1], and in elaborately institutionalized sodalities such as Poro for men and Sande for women.[2]

These sodalities initiate virtually all pubescent children into the first grade of adulthood, designating them "those who may procreate". They also sustain individuals in reproductive and economically productive activities throughout life. People with curiosity and ability rise to higher ranks commanding more knowledge and authority. At the end of mortal life, men in Poro, and women in Sande, are ceremonially carried through the final status transformation, into ancestorhood. The most valuable property these corporate sodalities have is their secret knowledge about successful reproduction, production and the continuity of social groups.

Puberty

In this area of West Africa first menstruation, marriage, defloration and birth of the first child are not important social ceremonies for a woman, but initiation into Sande at puberty is. Girls are initiated by older women in a class as small as three or four girls, to an occasional class of hundreds. The larger classes occur in ceremonies partly concerned with

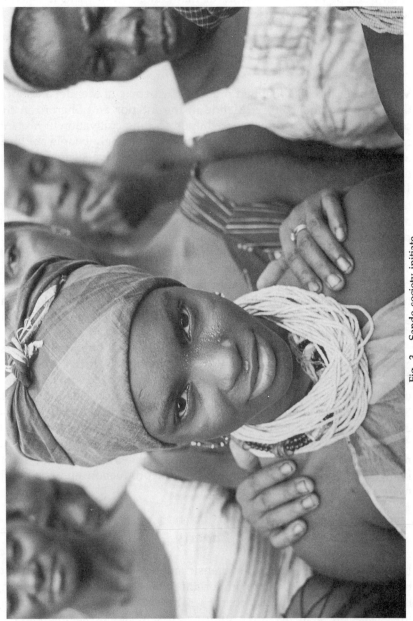

Fig. 3.   Sande society initiate.

the power of women in high political office (MacCormack, 1974, 1975). Initiations are held annually in populous areas, or as infrequently as every five years in small villages. In a large or an infrequently held class, girls may range in age from 8 to 17. These people are not interested in biological age, but in socially constructed age rankings. However, in conversations with nurse-midwives, we estimated that menarche is at about age 15, followed by a relatively short period of subfertility.

In the sequence of events in initiation ritual, girls first go through a portal, into a cleared place in the forest or a secluded compound in town, ritually separated from the social context in which they were girls. One of the most dramatic ritual elements they experience in their classic liminal state is clitoridectomy. The elderly head of the local chapter, who is usually midwife as well, excises the clitoris and part of the labia minora. Sande women explain that this makes women "clean". When invited to expand upon the meaning of "cleanness" in an attempt to gain insight into a folk model, Sande women commonly reply that a woman who is not initiated in this way will not be respected. No matter what her age, she will remain a girl socially while achieving womanhood biologically. At the level of the anthropologist's model, one might suggest a functionalist explanation that ritual scars or body modifications are signs that the person has been brought within a moral sphere. In this case, the man with whom a Sande woman shares an intimate relationship will know that she has been trained to the responsible role of potential procreator. At the level of structuralist explanation, "making women clean" removes the clitoris, the small male penis, making women fit unambiguously, purely and "cleanly" within the female category. Furthermore, the pain of clitoridectomy might be seen as a metaphor for childbirth itself.

The position assumed for clitoridectomy, on a mat on the ground, reclining against an older woman, often a kinswoman, is the same as the position assumed in childbirth. The place is the same, since ideally a woman returns to her natal initiation place to give birth, under the hand of the midwife who initiated her. The social group is similarly constituted of localized female kin and other townswomen, all being members of Sande. The pain of clitoridectomy, controlled by time, place and the technical skill of the midwife, is a metaphor for the pain of childbirth. As the midwife controls bleeding and protects against infection in clitoridectomy, so she does in childbirth. Womanhood is symbolically achieved in clitoridectomy and confirmed, under the midwife's hand, in childbirth. The two events are logically related as part of the same message, although they are separated in time (Douglas, 1966; Leach, 1976, pp. 25–27).

Nutrition and Fertility

The potential fertility of women is dependent upon such variables as age at puberty, neonatal mortality rate, the duration of lactational amenorrhoea and age at menopause (see Gray, 1979, p. 106 for other variables). These are mechanisms of population dynamics inherent in females, the "limiting resource" in human reproduction.

An important element in the ritual process of Sande initiation is fattening. Beauty, prosperity, health and fertility are explicitly linked to fatness, most graphically in the art which wells up from the Sande society. The opposite of fat is not thin, but dry, connoting among other things a dry and barren uterus. The liminal period of initiation lasts for a few weeks for some women, or two or three years for others. Bags of rice, gallons of palm oil, chickens and fish are sent into the initiation grove by kin of the initiates as part of the initiation fees. Not only the pubescent initiates, but mature Sande women as well, feast amid plenty. Frisch has noted that adolescent females go through a growth spurt which normally precedes menarche (1975, p. 319ff.). First ovulation, the actual commencement of a woman's fecund span, commences months or years after menarche (Short, 1976, p. 7; Kolata, 1974, p. 932). Frisch observed, in a sample of white North American girls, that the ratio of lean body weight to fat weight changes from 5:1 at the onset of the growth spurt to 3:1 at menarche. She suggests that a critical ratio of at least 20–22% fat, a minimal level of stored, easily metabolized energy for pregnancy and lactation, is required as a "safe guard" before regular ovulation occurs.

Undernutrition delays the growth spurt that increases the proportion of body fat while ample food advances it. Dickeman's tentative cross-cultural comparison suggests that fats and oils are most commonly inadequate in the diet of thin adolescents (1978). Indeed, it is the provision of generous quantities of palm oil that is stressed above all as a requirement for consumption in the Sande initiation grove. Mende and Sherbro girls are notably slim, but most take on the rounded contours characteristic of forest negro stock in adolescence. Throughout their adult life women are especially proud of their full, rounded buttocks, displayed to advantage in the way they tie their clothes, and in dance. Women often dance together in a group, displaying full rounded contours in a message of fecundity and social power as producers and reproducers.

If we assume that ritual adolescent fattening is a cultural strategy, on an unconscious level, for early fecundity, then in a comparative sense these rural Mende and Sherbro people are doing rather well in

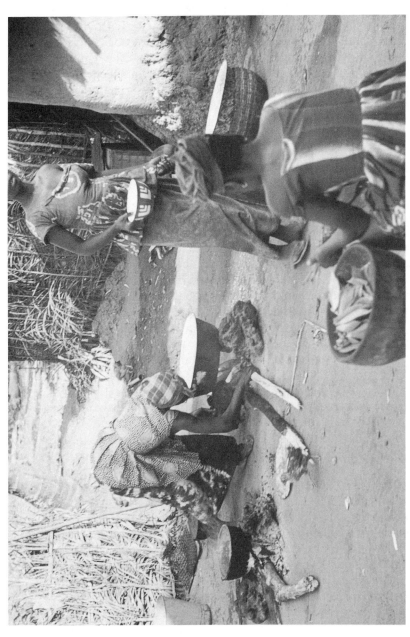

Fig. 4. Women cooking. Green leaves, said to be good for the blood, are in the foreground, palm oil is in the pan on the fire.

achieving menarche by about age 15. Recent mean age of menarche in affluent countries is 12.4 to 13.5 years (Marshall and Tanner, 1974). Mean age of menarche in India is 13 to 14 years, 15 years in South African Bantu speaking populations, 15.7 in Bangladesh and 18.8 years for the poorly nourished Bundi women of Papua New Guinea. Sixteen years is estimated as the age of menarche for nineteenth century Europe. These are mean figures, perhaps reflecting an urban bias. Differences of a few months to about two years have been measured between urban and rural populations in the same society, and differences of up to two years for girls in varying social classes in the United States (Bongaarts, 1979, pp. 8–9).

Unfortunately, I was not able to obtain a reliable estimate of biological age of menopause. From observing the onset of weight loss with aging, my "hunch" is that women are well nourished, experience relatively late menopause and have a long span of potential fecundity compared with other populations in developing countries (see Gray, 1979). Assuming that nutrition and age of menopause are related, women's nutritional status depends upon a number of social variables. In Sierra Leone land is not scarce, nor has it been made artificially scarce through privatization of land holding. In rural southern Sierra Leone land is the corporate estate of descent groups and every married woman has the right to use farm land of her natal cognatic descent group and/or her husband's group. The residential compound, averaging ten people, farms as a cooperative labour unit and a head wife is as likely to keep the key to the granary as is her husband (49% of wives, 51% of husbands retained the key). Furthermore, women can make their own farms, market gardens, or make palm oil and other products which they either retain, exchange, or market.

Women's nutritional status and fecundity also depends upon patterns of birth spacing and lactation. Mende and Sherbo women breast-feed for about 12 to 18 months. The baby is carried on its mother's back by day and sleeps with her by night suckling on demand over the entire diurnal cycle. The Sande society also enforces a postpartum taboo on sexual intercourse while the mother lactates, and will publicly fine anyone who violates this ancestral law. Long postpartum taboos, a kind of cultural contraception, are particularly associated with societies having an economy based upon land extensive agriculture (Saucier, 1972), as indeed typifies the Mende and Sherbro economies.

In addition to abstenance, contraception is also associated with lactation itself in a way which is not fully understood in Western medicine. Nutritional status of the lactating mother is part of the picture, as is frequency and vigour of sucking. Frisch (1978) has suggested that poorly nourished lactating women are simply thin, and their menstrual cycles will resume when fat again composes at least 22% of body weight. This might be the case where women are so poor that they are malnourished in the third trimester of pregnancy and unable to increase food consumption to compensate for the requirements of pregnancy and lactation, but should they become better nourished, or should their infant be given supplementary food, the frequency of breast-feeding draining will diminish, and the woman may regain the fat necessary to trigger the hormonal reflex system for commencing menstruation and ovulation (Delgado *et al.*, 1978, p. 323; Delgado *et al.*, 1979, p. 306; Lunn *et al.*, 1980, p. 623).

This hypothesis has been tested on a sample of 2048 women at the Cholera Research Laboratory in Bangladesh. The effect of nutrition on length of lactational amenorrhoea seems negligible: 17.9 months for poorly nourished women and 16.8 months for well nourished women (Huffman *et al.*, 1978a, pp. 1155-1156; 1978b; Gray, 1980, p. 1026). In Guatemala, undernourished women had amenorrhoea for 14.8 months and better nourished women had it for 13.2 months. We might conclude then that poor women may breast-feed as long as possible because they lack appropriate weaning foods, and mothers' nutritional differentials only account for 1–1.5 months of additional infertility, a small fraction of the birth interval which is generally 2 to 3 years (Gray, 1980, p. 1026).

Another important factor is frequency and intensity of infant suckling which may have an effect by inducing surges of prolactin which inhibits ovulation (Short, 1974; Delvoye *et al.*, 1977; Huffman *et al.*, 1978a, p. 1157; Delgado, 1978, p. 325). These two hypotheses are related in that supplementary infant feeding decreases the duration and intensity of suckling.

In regard to Mende and Sherbro mothers, we might conclude that children are successfully spaced because of cultural rules, taught and enforced through the Sande society: that (1) lactating women must not have sexual intercourse and (2) women must comfort and put their infant to the breast whenever it shows distress, until the weaning crisis before age two. There is potential for helpful Western medical advice on appropriate weaning foods to improve child health, but maternal health, based upon good intake of carbohydrates, vegetable oils, leaves, vegetables, fruit and some protein, is rather good.

Deliberate adolescent fattening, and beliefs about the beauty of full-bodied mature women, is undoubtedly of selective advantage in populations which experience seasonality in food supply. Indeed, Sierra Leone has a marked dry season when crops are harvested and food is plentiful, contrasted with a wet season when granary stocks are low and maximum farm labour is needed. Better maternal nutrition is also adaptive in that well fed mothers tend to have larger babies with better survival chances, especially if the babies weigh more than 2.5kg (Habicht *et al.*, 1974).

In summary, deliberate ritual adolescent fattening can advance the age of menarche, can "confer" fertility, enhance the survival chances of babies born to those well nourished women and guard the health of the women themselves.

Folk Meanings of Fertility

When Sherbro and Mende women speak of health, fertility and child-bearing, they say they speak "women's words". The words themselves are often common words, used by both men and women, but the concepts they stand for have come from women's experience in ancestral time. Many of the words are polysemous, allowing women to speak in punning riddles. For example, "water" means, among other things, semen, amniotic fluid and the underneath part of the cosmos, the abode of ancestors. Drinks used for libations are called "cold water", and poured out upon the ground they mediate between the living and the watery underworld of ancestors. Being in a liminal stage in Sande society initiation, being physically in the initiation grove, is being "under water". Seeds germinate in water. In the initiation grove ancestral information is imparted which allows a woman's fertility to root and flower. The foetus within a woman is "stone", again polysemous, as a cobble under river water, or a cherry stone, or the kernel of an avocado. Childbirth is pulling stone out of water.

Within Sande there is a sub-group of women who keep the bird laws (Boone, 1978). They are pregnant women, but since a woman does not always know when she is pregnant, some always keep the laws. A principal law is not to eat bird and especially not to eat eggs. Birds mediate between the sky of an otiose creator god and the earth of mundane humans. They also go under water, the cosmological realm of ancestors and ancestresses. Domestic fowl are found at the margins of the compound, or of the village, and symbolize the ability to know future events, detecting the approach of strangers before the people of the village know of their approach. Wild birds in tree tops similarly "see" the future. One of the most powerful Sande midwives in Moyamba District was renowned for her ability to transcend time and space in her command of knowledge.

Birds have qualities which fertile, nurturing, "complete" women have: they rise early, are cheerfully active through the day, shelter and protect their young, build nests, find food, sing beautifully and sleep at night. The reverse of this goodness is nocturnal birds, particularly the owl and the fruit bat, which do not sleep at night but are transformations of evil persons ruled by greed and envy. They are witches in the black of night, opposed to the light of day.

Some of the leaves which diurnal domestic fowl favour constitute important "medicines" for pregnant women. "Medicine", *hale* in Mende and *nrom* in Sherbro, is a unitary concept which we tend to split apart into three separate concepts: plants with an inherent potency based upon their pharmacological properties, plants which have been ritually energized with supernatural power directed to a specific end and plants which evoke a metaphoric relationship between their own qualities and a desired result. Medicine in the first category might be leaves rich in iron which women eat to build their blood. Many of the greens women cook into palm oil sauces are consciously chosen because, women say, they are good for the blood. Or, the leaves of the Saville orange, *Citrus aurantium*, are boiled and the liquid drunk as a diuretic when swelling and other signs of pre-eclampsia are detected. There are also medicines to induce contractions, stop contractions, stop bleeding and so forth. Most are crushed in water, or boiled in water, and the liquid is drunk. Some, such as *Ageratum conyzoides*, are crushed in the hands with water and the juice instilled into the vagina to clot blood quickly. At least two alternative plants are used as a vaginal lubricant to facilitate birth. One way of increasing a lactating woman's milk is to steam the breasts over medicated vapours. (A list of medicines and their uses is appended.)

In the second category are various plants which have been ritually transformed into amulets or other objects which protect the pregnant woman. For example, bark from the tree *Bussea occidentalis* is worn on a black and white cord around the waist to protect a woman from the envy and malice of those who might wish her to abort; to protect her from witches (Kargbo, 1975, p. 3).

Some food prohibitions illustrate the metaphoric concepts of medicine. For example, a pregnant woman must not eat the electric fish, *Gymnarchus niloticus*, which may cause tetanus in the new-born child. The muscle contractions stimulated by contact with the fish are analogous to the spasms caused by the disease. If a pregnant woman stands in the doorway she may cause her own obstructed labour, or if she stands at crossroads she may cause the foetus to assume a transverse lie position. Other avoidances are more pragmatic. Heavy work or lifting heavy loads may cause a woman to abort. However, if a woman is too inactive in pregnancy the uterus may become inert. (A further list of avoidances is appended.)

For the Sherbro, with a cognatic descent system, both husband and wife complementarily contribute to the growth of the foetus. Some plants used in pregnancy are considered to be female, others are male. A leaf named *tot* in Sherbro, from a female vine, is brewed and the liquid drunk early in pregnancy to strengthen the foetus. A leaf, similar in appearance, named *tote*, from a male vine, is brewed and the liquid drunk late in pregnancy to strengthen the uterus.

Birth

Onset of labour is observed from hardening of the uterus and rhythmic contractions. In normal delivery, the woman reclines on a mat supported by an older woman. Her hands are washed with cold water from an earthen pot. She may be given medicine to strengthen contractions, the medicine made from crushing either *Ficus exasperata* or *Carica papaya* leaves in water, and the liquid is drunk.

When the woman is ready to push she tells the midwife that she wants to defecate. The midwife looks for the baby's head, and if she does not see it, she will wash her hands and do a vaginal examination to feel for the head. Commonly, the woman in the last stages of birth squats on a mat, the position for defecation, and pushes the baby out. Or, if she is tired, she may recline against another woman. In this position, the midwife presses her toe on the perineum while the woman is pushing, supporting the perineum to keep it from tearing as the baby is born. The umbilical cord is cut after the placenta is expelled.

The baby's cord is tied with locally spun cotton and cut with the edge of a sharp leaf of a sedge, *Cyperus rotundus*, or with razor blade, knife, scissors or other sharp object. The severed cord is dressed with *Bryophyllum pinnatum*, called "never-die leaf", until it drops. Alternatively, it may be dressed with *Xylopia aethiopica*, a spice which is ground with a few drops of water, or chewed kola nuts, *Cola nitida*, or tobacco leaf, *Nicotiana tabacum*, or the dirt in the bottom of earthen drinking pots, or the juice squeezed from banana shoots. Medication is renewed daily until the cord drops off.

If labour is difficult, lasting more than two days, the cause is sought. Had she had sexual intercourse with someone other than her husband? Since both husband and wife contribute to the substance of the foetus, another man's contribution would be anomalous. She must confess to clear the obstruction. Had anyone with a grievance exercised witchcraft against her? A diviner is consulted and the aggrieved person thus identified is begged to perform a ceremony of forgiveness. He or she holds a glass of water, says words of forgiveness to the patient, gargles water, spits it on the ground, and the resulting mud is rubbed on the woman's abdomen from sternum to umbilicus. The remaining water is spat upon her abdomen (Kargbo, 1975, p. 8).

If the woman still fails to deliver, the midwife will exercise her judgement on the basis of presentation. With a head presentation, the midwife sits astride the patient's chest and performs fundal pressure. A stick across the abdomen may be used to apply more pressure, with the danger of uterine rupture. An object may be stuck in her mouth to encourage her to cough the baby out. A second midwife may stretch the vagina upward while pressing the perineum downward with her toe.

With breach presentation the baby is lubricated with palm oil and the legs of the baby are lifted up toward the mother. If this fails, then the midwife must pull with force.

With transverse lie, the woman is given a hot bath or hot palm oil is put on her abdomen as she lies on her side facing the fire. The heated abdomen may stimulate the baby to turn. If the baby does not turn, the suspicion may grow that the mother herself may be culpable. She may have stood at crossroads, or committed a more deliberate wrong. The husband may be able to help. A piece of tobacco leaf is sent to him to report the difficult labour. Possibly his wife had peeped at the masked spirit of the men's society, and her husband then pours libations to that spirit to allow her to deliver.

If the baby is abnormal at birth, it is socially defined as the incarnation of a malevolent spirit. The mother is prevented from feeding it, and it is left to die.

Throughout a normal childbirth the woman receives considerable social support from Sande women, just as she did during clitoridectomy. However, should a difficult birth continue until all hope is lost, social support is withdrawn from her. The fault must be the woman's. It cannot be Sande's. Thus her failure to deliver is attributed to her own dark side, where she secretly practised witchcraft or other social evils. She loses the sympathy of her Sande "sisters", her husband, her parents and other kin. In a last desperate attempt to save herself she may confess to causing deaths and poor harvests through witchcraft.

Mortality

Neonatal tetanus is a major cause of infant mortality. Taking up only one of several possible causes, the banana grows in kitchen gardens, at the rear of a residential compound. All household refuse, including animal droppings, are swept or thrown there. Goats, sheep, pigs and chickens forage there for food. A banana shoot comes off the stem below ground, in contact with the debris around the tree base. The infant may be infected on the day of birth or any subsequent day the cord is dressed. The first symptom mothers detect, appearing in the fifth to ninth day of life, is the baby's inability to suck, followed by muscle spasms (Wilkinson, 1961, p.2ff.). Sande practitioners have medicines to treat tetanus, but I do not know how they affect the infants' survival chances.

Some women lose baby after baby. There is not a consistent Mende or Sherbro belief concerning reincarnation. Some people believe that a person at death is transmuted into another person (Boone, 1978). Those children "born to die" in a cycle of reincarnation are called by the words meaning "rubbish" or "garbage", the trash in the kitchen garden out of which something new grows. The "troublesome" dead infant may be buried in that rubbish heap.

Genetically-linked diseases may also explain in part the tendency for some women to be particularly unlucky in their efforts to keep their children alive; in giving birth to children "born to die". Sickle cell anaemia provides an example. Carriers of the haemoglobin sickle cell trait have enhanced protection against death from *Plasmodium falciparum* malaria. People with the sickling trait are thought to be as easily infected as any others, but the parasites, in their active feeding stage, multiply less quickly than in a person with normal haemoglobin. Duration of illness appears to be shorter, incidence of cerebral malaria lower and mortality lower (Dacie, 1960, pp. 250-251). The selective advantage in having the sickling trait is for children between the ages of four and six months, when they lose the protection of foetal haemoglobin, and have not yet acquired some immunity to malaria (Lehman and Huntsman, 1974, p. 144; Dacie, 1960, p. 250; Serjeant, 1974, pp. 30–32). It is the heterozygotes, with both Haemoglobin A (normal adult haemoglobin) and Haemoglobin S (with sickle haemoglobin) who enjoy this selective advantage. Most homozygotes, for Haemoglobin S only, die of sickle cell anaemia. Dacie reports that in a sample of infants in Central Africa with sickle cell disease, half died within the first year of life. Only 2 in 244 reached adulthood. In equatorial Africa the prevalence of the sickle cell trait is as high as 40% of the adult population (Serjeant, 1974, p. 28). In the Mende area of Sierra Leone, about 30.6% of a sample had the trait (Rose and Suliman, 1955).

With a prevalence of 30.6% in the adult population, the probability that the father has the trait is about 0.3, and the probability that the mother has the trait is also 0.3. Assuming that mating is independent of genotype, the probability that both parents have the trait is the product of the above two numbers, or 0.09 (9%). In Africa, if both should have the trait, then the probability for each of their children is 1:4 that they will be homozygous and die. Therefore, in the total population there is about a 2% probability that any birth will be homozygous.

$$0.3 \times 0.3 = 0.09$$
$$0.09 \times 0.25 = 0.02$$

But what Mende and Sherbro systems of explanation are concerned with is misfortune within *families:* "Why do *our* children die?" If both mother and father have the sickling trait, then the probability of a homozygous child being born rises to 25%. When risk from neonatal tetanus, diarrhoeal diseases and other hazards are added to the calculation, child mortality rates in some families could be very high indeed.[3]

Sickle cell disease is recognized as a distinct disease category and named in the indigenous languages of West African people (Konotey-Ahulu, 1968). Symptoms commonly appear between the ages of three months and two years. The syndrome Sande practitioners especially note is the painful swelling of one or more hands or feet. They treat sickle cell disease with plant medicines just as they medicate for neonatal tetanus. They are definitely more successful with some diseases than with others. They also treat the social and psychological roots of illness. A single practitioner combines and integrates chemical therapy with psychological and social therapy.

Conclusion

The conceptual framework within which senior Sande women work is very broad and flexible, not at all the closed system which Horton has suggested in his discussions of African thought (Horton, 1974, p. 153ff.). Midwives have readily shown me their stainless steel scissors which they now know are free from contamination and will diminish the chances of neonatal tetanus. They have much to gain by adopting new theoretical tenets about health and fertility in order to improve their own success, fame and power.

Witchcraft, however, is still very much a part of the conceptual framework of childbirth, for the reason Evans-Pritchard suggested at least 40 years ago. The Mende, Sherbro, and indeed the Zande, often know the physical causes of disease or difficult birth. But witchcraft explains why a particular woman and no other suffered. Why did Boema die in childbirth when Yema's baby was "pulled" smoothly? Witchcraft provides the causal link which makes a more satisfying explanation.

Evans-Pritchard attempted rather unsatisfactorily to make a distinction between Zande medicines which were either mystical or empirically efficacious. One Sherbro medicine, for example, is compounded from parts of 14 plants. Some undoubtedly have empirically proven pharmacological properties, an inherent potency, and others fulfil "mediating" functions. They facilitate the metaphorical transfer of the qualities of some plants into the qualities desired in the patient.

Tambiah (1973) has shown us a way around Evans-Pritchard's false dichotomy between magical thought and scientific thought. Both are analogical thought. Reasoning by analogy has always been a characteristic of human thought. Analogy depends on the recognition of similarities, a process of reasoning from experience to the conceptualization of a particular problem. Magical thought results in "performative" acts which seek to transfer imperatively a property in nature (e.g. the strong "never die" leaf) to a recipient (e.g. the umbilical stump of a new-born child). The transfer of qualities is made on an analogical basis; the leaf may be ritually placed upon the umbilicus as a spell is said: "child live long, as this leaf does". Analogy may also be used to evoke attitudes, as in the following example used by Tambiah

father : employer
child : worker.

In scientific thought, analogy is used more to predict than to evoke. A sample is tested and measured to serve as a model for the remainder of the phenomenon to be explained. The model is used to generate a prediction about the total phenomenon. In this way, we reason by analogy to discover natural causes and predict empirical consequences. The adequacy of the model is judged by inductive rules and tests of falsifiability, while the adequacy of analogy in magical thought is judged by its ability to persuade or offer satisfactory conceptualization. For Mende and Sherbro people both kinds of analogical thought are part of a single conceptual system which explains health, fertility and birth in coastal southern Sierra Leone. These thought systems, together with the social systems of the Sande society and other sodalities, are the foundation upon which an effective primary health care system might be built. A "top down" plan based upon Western medical thought alone would be unfortunate.

Notes

(1) Descent groups are cognatic for the Sherbro, and patrilineal with some cognatic tendencies for the Mende.

(2) Sande is also known by the Temne and Krio term *Bundu*. In the Sherbro language it is *Bondo*. See MacCormack (1979) and Little (1965, 1966) for further details of Sande and Poro.

(3) Infant and child mortality as a World Health Organization indicator of progress towards health for all by the year 2000 must take into account these genetic traits. They are adaptive at one level of analysis, but maladaptive if the focus is only child deaths. Populations with these genetic characteristics are unlikely to equal the child mortality statistics of populations without them.

(4) Information is from author's field notes and Kargbo (1975). Botanical terms are in agreement with Dalziel (1937). For description of birth practices and medicines in the nearby Mano area of Liberia, see Harley (1970).

References

Bongaarts, J. (1979). *Malnutrition and Fecundity: A Summary of Evidence.* Center for Policies Studies Working Paper No. 51. New York: The Population Council.

Boone, S. (1978). Personal communication. New Haven: Yale University Department of Fine Arts.

Dacie, J. V. (1960). *The Haemolytic Anaemias.* Second edition. London: Churchill.

Dalziel, J. M. (1937). *The Useful Plants of West Tropical Africa.* London: Crown Agents.

Dapper, O. (1964) [1668]. "Umbstaendliche und Eigentliche Beschreibung von Africa". In *Sierra Leone Inheritance* (C. Fyfe, ed.), pp. 35–40. Oxford: Oxford University Press.

Delgado, H., Lechtig, A., Martorell, R., Brineman, E. and Klein, R. (1978). "Nutrition, Lactation and Postpartum Amenorrhea". *American Journal of Clinical Nutrition* **31**, 322–327.

Delgado, H., Lechtig, A., Martorell, R., Brineman, E. and Klein, R. (1979). "Effects of Maternal Nutritional Status on Infant Supplementation During Lactation in Postpartum Amenorrhea". *American Journal of Obstetrics and Gynecology* **135**, 303–307.

Delvoye, P., Demaegd, M., Desnoeck-Delogne, J. and Robyn, C. (1977). "The Influence of the Frequency of Nursing and of Previous Lactation Experience on Serum Prolactin in Lactating Mothers". *Journal of Biosocial Science* **9**, 447–451.

Dickeman, M. (1978). Personal communication. Rohnerts Park, California: Sonoma State College.

Douglas, M. (1966). *Purity and Danger*. London: Routledge and Kegan Paul.

Dow, T. E. (1972). "Fertility and Family Planning in Sierra Leone". *Studies in Family Planning* **2**, 153–165.

Evans-Pritchard, E. E. (1937). *Witchcraft, Oracles and Magic among the Azande*. Oxford: Clarendon Press.

Frisch, R. E. (1975). "Critical Weight, a Critical Body Composition, Menarche, and the Maintenance of Menstrual Cycles". In *Biosocial Interrelations in Population Adaption* (E. S. Watts, F. E. Johnston and G. W. Lasker, eds), pp. 319–352. The Hague: Mouton.

Frisch, R. E. (1978). "Population, Food Intake and Fertility". *Science* **119**, 22.

Gray, R. H. (1979). "Biological and Social Interactions in the Determination of Late Fertility". *Journal of Biosocial Science*, Suppl. 6, 97–115.

Gray, R. H. (1980). "Maternal Diet and Prolactin". *Lancet*, May 10, 1980, 1026–1027.

Habicht, J.-P., Lechtig, A., Yarbrough, C. and Klein, R. E. (1974). "Maternal Nutrition, Birth Weight and Infant Mortality". In *Size at Birth*, CIBA Foundation Symposium 27, pp. 353–377. Amsterdam: Elsevier.

Harley, G. W. (1970) [1941]. *Native African Medicine with Special Reference to its Practice in the Mano Tribe of Liberia*. London: Frank Cass.

Horton, R. (1974). "African Traditional Thought and Western Science". In *Rationality* (B. R. Wilson, ed.), pp. 131–171. Oxford: Basil Blackwell.

Huffman, S. L., Alauddin Chowdhury, A. K. M. and Mosley, W. H. (1978a). "Postpartum Amenorrhea: How is it Affected by Maternal Nutritional Status?" *Science* **200**, 1155–1157.

Huffman, S. L., Alauddin Chowdhury, A. K. M. and Mosley, W. H. (1978b). "Nutrition and Postpartum Amenorrhoea in Rural Bangladesh". *Population Studies* **32**, 251–260.

Kargbo, T. K. (1975). *Traditional Midwifery Amongst the Mende of the Southern Province of Sierra Leone*. Freetown: Fourah Bay College. Mimeograph.

Kolata, G. B. (1974). "!Kung Hunter-Gatherers, Feminism, Diet and Birth Control". *Science* **185**, 932–934.

Konotey-Ahulu, F. I. D. (1968). "Hereditary Qualitative and Quantitative Erythrocyte Defects in Ghana: an Historical and Geographical Survey". *Ghana Medical Journal* **7**, 118.

Leach, E. R. (1976). *Culture and Communication*. Cambridge: Cambridge University Press.

Lehmann, H. and Huntsman, R. G. (1974). *Man's Haemoglobins*. Amsterdam: North Holland Publishing.

Little, K. (1965, 1966). "The Political Function of the Poro", Parts I and II. *Africa* **35**, 349–365, **36**, 62–71.

Lunn, P. G., Prentice, A. M., Austin, S. and Whitehead, R. G. (1980). "Influence of Maternal Diet on Plasma-Prolactin Levels During Lactation". *Lancet*, March 22, 1980, 623–625.

MacCormack (Hoffer), C. P. (1972). "Mende and Sherbro Women in High Office". *Canadian Journal of African Studies* **6**, 151–164.

MacCormack, C. P. (1974). "Madam Yoko: Ruler of the Kpa Mende Confederacy". In *Woman Culture and Society* (M. Z. Rosaldo and L. Lamphere, eds), pp. 173–187. Stanford: Stanford University Press.

MacCormack, C. P. (1975). "Sande Women and Political Power in Sierra Leone". *West African Journal of Sociology and Political Science* **1**, 42–50.

MacCormack, C. P. (1978)."The Cultural Ecology of Production: Sherbro Coast and Hinterland". In *Social Organization and Settlement* (D. Green, C. Haselgrove and M. Spriggs, eds) Oxford: British Archaeological Reports.

MacCormack, C. P. (1979). "Sande: the Public Face of a Secret Society". In *The New Religions of Africa* (B. Jules-Rosette, ed.). Norwood, N.J.: Ablex.

MacCormack, C. P. (1981). "Proto-social to Adult: A Sherbro Transformation". In *Nature Culture and Gender* (C. P. MacCormack and M. Strathern, eds). Cambridge: Cambridge University Press.

Margai, M. A. S. (1948). "Welfare Work in a Secret Society". *African Affairs* **47**, 227–230.

Marshall, W. A. and Tanner, J. M. (1974). "Puberty". In *Scientific Foundations of Paediatrics* (J. A. Davis and J. Dobbing, eds). London: Heinemann.

Minette, N. (1980). Personal communication. Freetown: CARE.

Rose, J. R. and Suliman, J. K. (1955). "The Sickle Cell Trait in the Mende Tribe of Sierra Leone". *West African Medical Journal* **4**, 35.

Saucier, J.-F. (1972). "Correlates of the Long Postpartum Taboo: A Cross-Cultural Study". *Current Anthropology* **13**, 238–249.

Serjeant, G. R. (1974). *The Clinical Features of Sickle Cell Disease*. Amsterdam: North Holland Publishing.

Short, R. V. (1976). "The Evolution of Human Reproduction". In *Contraceptives of the Future*. A Royal Society Discussion, pp. 3–24. London: The Royal Society.

Tambiah, J. S. (1973). "Form and Meaning in Magical Acts: A Point of View". In *Modes of Thought* (R. Horton and R. Finnegan, eds), pp. 199–229. London: Faber and Faber.

Wilkinson, J. L. (1961). "Neonatal Tetanus in Sierra Leone". *British Medical Journal* **1**, 1721–1724.

Appendix[4]

Avoidances

Foods avoided in pregnancy:

Eggs and chicken. See text. They also cause diarrhoea in the infant.

Fish. Causes mucus in infants.

Electric fish, *Gymnarchus niloticus*. Causes tetanus.

Beans. Causes the umbilical cord to wrap around baby's neck.

Plantain, *Musa sapientum*. Causes placenta to be retained, or causes large phallus in male infant.

Intestine of animals. Causes abnormal skin pigmentation.

Brain of animals. Causes infection of inner ear.

Garden eggs, *Solanum incanum*. Causes pemphigus.

Coconut, *Cocos nucifera*. May cause antepartum haemorrhage or heavy postpartum haemorrhage.

Activities avoided in pregnancy:

Taking purgative herbs such as *Morinda geminata*. This herb is used as an abortifacient. It is also used as a laxative, and its root is used for fever.

Lifting heavy loads, fishing for a long time (with hand net), washing heavy clothes such as cotton blankets. Causes abortion or premature labour.

Not moving about in pregnancy. Causes uterus to become inert.

Frequent intercourse, and especially intercourse with a man other than husband. Causes abortion, antepartum haemorrhage, premature labour or difficult birth.

Erotic dreams. If a woman dreams she is having intercourse with another man resembling her husband it is witchcraft. If she has erotic dreams about a man different from her husband it is spirits of the wild.

Wearing brassiere, or wrapping the lappa (dressing cloth) around the neck rather than the waist. Causes the umbilical cord to wrap around baby's neck.

Standing at cross roads. Transverse lie presentation.

Using pit latrine. Buttocks presentation.

Lying on an easy chair, hammock, or intruding noisily in other people's affairs. Face presentation.

Laying fire with old firewood placed in the wrong way. Footling breach.

Walking at night without a knife tied in the lappa for protection. Footling breach or abnormal baby.

Bathing or defecating outdoors at night. Will be seen by spirits of the wild causing abnormal baby.

Standing in doorway. Obstructed labour.

Setting out on journey with headload and returning to collect forgotten item. Difficult labour.

Medicines

Antenatal, pre-eclampsia and eclampsia:

A paper amulet sewn into leather sachet, called *sebe* (Mende), is worn around the neck during pregnancy as a preventative measure to drive away spirits and witchcraft which cause this disease.

Dialium guineense (Mende: *Mamboi*) or black tamarind. The strong and young leaves are ground with water and mixed with the calyx of *Hibiscus sabdariffa* (Mende: *Satoi*) which has been boiled in water.

This mixture is drunk as a diuretic at the early signs of eclampsia. A woman's swelling feet are taken as a sign of foetal maturity.

Citris aurantium (Mende: *Dumbele*) or Seville orange. Leaves are boiled and liquid is drunk as a diuretic.

Capsicum species (Mende: *Pujei*) or pepper. Small leaves are rubbed in the hand and the juice is instilled into the woman's eyes for eclampsia fits. The cause of fits is attributed to spirits and a strong Muslim man is called to give treatment.

Antenatal bleeding:

Bertiera spicata (Mende: *Kafa-hinei*). The young leaves are ground with water, salt and palm oil. Incantations about the pregnancy are said while mixing the ingredients. The mixture is then drunk by the bleeding woman.

Dialium guineense (Mende: *Mamboi*) or black tamarind. The young leaves are ground on a stone with some salt and eaten.

Lindackeria dentata (Mende: *Toya-hinei*). Tender leaves are rubbed in a calabash with water and liquid is drunk.

Newbouldia laevis (Mende: *Poma magbe*). Bark of trunk and roots is ground on a stone with water and liquid is drunk.

Tetracera alnifolia (Mende: *Katata-wai*). Leaves are ground with water and liquid is drunk.

Gouania longipetala (Mende: *Sawa-wai*). There may be two varieties of this. One grows on the ground and stops bleeding. The other grows on the trees and is used to stop contractions. The tender leaves are ground in a calabash with water and the slimy liquid is drunk.

Spondias monbin (Mende: *Kpoji laa*). Leaves are boiled and liquid is drunk.

Ageratum conyzoides (Mende: *Yonigbei*). The leaves are crushed in the hands with water and the juice is instilled in the vagina to clot blood quickly.

Wash face with coconut water and drink some.

Sit on an old fishing net.

Antenatal contractions:

Banana stalk is squeezed and liquid is drunk by woman.

Microdesmis puberula (Mende: *Kikili*). Leaves are ground with water, the liquid is drunk and crushed leaves are rubbed on the head.

Desmodium species (Mende: *Nanei*). Young leaves are ground with water and liquid is drunk.

Diarrhoea (may be caused by eating too much, or "dirty" stomach):
  Palm oil from *Elaeis guineensis* is heated and about 2 oz drunk.
  Ficus species (Mende: *Kponi*), fig. Leaves are ground with salt, water
    is added, and liquid is drunk.
  Morinda geminata (Mende: *Nsa-suwi*). Boiled and liquid drunk.

Labour:
  Hibiscus sabdariffa (Mende: *Satui*), red sorrel or sour-sour.
  Leaves are boiled and liquid is drunk to induce contractions. It is also
    used as a diuretic.
  Necepsia species? (Mende: *Yumbuyambei*), Sierra Leone peach. Roots
    are boiled and liquid is drunk to induce contractions. Also used
    as a purgative.
  Carica papaya (Mende: *Fakali*), papaw. Old yellow leaves are ground
    in a calabash with water and liquid is drunk to increase contractions.
  Ficus exasperata (Mende: *Magumbu*). Leaves ground in a small pot
    with a little water and liquid is drunk to increase contractions.
    Some is rubbed on the abdomen.
  Urera species (Mende: *Ndogbo yaingeh*). Leaves are ground and be-
    come very slimy. Water is added, and mixture is used as a vaginal
    lubricant to facilitate birth.

Retained placenta:
  Xylopia aethiopica (Mende: *Hewei*). The spice is boiled and liquid is
    given to mother to drink. The cord is tied to head of an axe to
    apply constant pressure. *Hewei* contracts the uterus while axe head
    applies pressure.
  Ocimum viride (Mende: *Kumulu*), fever plant or tea bush. Leaves are
    crushed with water and liquid is drunk. This is also given for fever.
  Woman squats and pushes to expel placenta.
  Woman is knocked on head with husband's shoe or any man's shoe.
  A piece of cloth is tied around the ribs to prevent the placenta from
    going up to the heart and chest.

Umbilical cord:
  Cyperus rotundus (Mende: *Njawa-wa*), a type of sedge. Sharp leaf is
    used to cut the umbilical cord.
  Bryophyllum pinnatum (Mende: *Kpowolaa*), never-die leaf. Leaf is used
    to dress the cord until the cord drops off.
  Xylopia aethiopica (Mende: *Hewei*). The spice is ground with a few
    drops of water and rubbed on the cord. Chewed kola (*Cola nitida*)
    or tobacco (*Nicotiana tabacum*) may also be applied.

Postpartum haemorrhage:
   Tetracera alnifolia (Mende: *Ndopa nei*). Leaves crushed and liquid is
   drunk.

Care of infant:
   Green palm kernels, *Elaeis guineensis* (Mende: *Towui*) are boiled with
   water and the baby is bathed in the liquid. Moisture is left to
   evaporate from the baby's body.
   The bark of the fig, *Ficus* species (Mende: *Kponeh*) is cut from the
   eastern and western flanks and boiled in water. Baby is bathed in
   water and given some to drink. Moisture is left to evaporate from
   the baby's body. It makes the baby gain weight and prevents
   constipation.
   Newbouldia laevis (Mende: *Pomamagbei*) roots are washed, scraped, cut
   in small pieces and boiled in water. Baby is bathed in the liquid
   and moisture is left to evaporate.
   Herbs or scraped bark are mixed with palm oil and rubbed on the
   baby's body.

5. Interpretations of Infertility: the Aowin People of South-west Ghana

V. EBIN

Introduction

This paper examines the interpretations of infertility provided by two different types of healers among the Aowin people of south-west Ghana. We look first at the explanations and treatment dispensed by the female spirit mediums and contrast this with the views held by the male herbalists.

The Aowins are a matrilineal people whose political and social organization closely resembles that of the neighbouring Asante (see Busia, 1954; Fortes, 1950; Rattray, 1923). They have a hierarchical political structure in which judicial and ritual authority is focussed in the office of the paramount chief, the Omanhene, who has his court in Enchi, the principal town in the Aowin state. Here he carries out his official duties with the help of the other members of his court, the Queen Mother, the village chiefs, the court linguists through whom he speaks on official occasions and the spirit mediums. In Enchi there are 13 mediums and at this time they all are women. They are responsible for mediating between the Aowins and the spirit world and it is their official duty to maintain the well-being of the town; in times of crisis, epidemics and heavy rains, the Omanhene calls upon them to perform the communal ritual, known as the *momome*. In this rite they sweep the streets of the town and outline its borders in white clay. They define the boundaries between the town and the forest and in this way

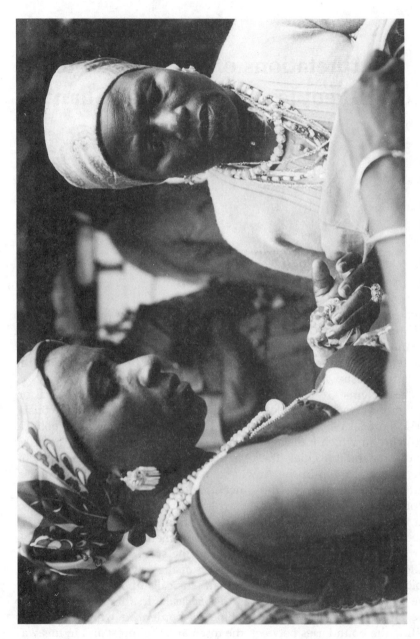

Fig. 1. Priestess prepares white clay for the purification ritual.

express the polarity between the social universe and the world of mystical power. A harmonious relationship between men and the spirits depends on maintaining these boundaries. The mediums also enforce certain practices such as the use of space within the town, the observance of the sacred days and ritual prohibitions which form the pattern of everyday life. The mediums carry out these duties under the supervision of a head medium who is appointed by the Omanhene. She has a special position at the Omanhene's court, equivalent to that of a sub-chief, and she is allowed to use the symbols of power, usually associated with chieftaincy: the gold regalia, drums and linguist staffs. These staffs which are carved in wood and covered with gold leaf often represent Ashanti proverbs which refer to the power of the chief. A medium may be possessed by a royal ancestor or by the chief god of the Aowin pantheon (who holds a position among the gods equivalent to the Omanhene). On these occasions, the medium in her possessed state represents the identity of her god by displaying the appropriate accessories: the large sandals worn by chiefs, the style of cloth and, as the chief god, she is served by another medium who represents another god identified as a court linguist.

In addition to their official role, the mediums also act as individual practitioners and are asked for their diagnosis and treatment of illness and affliction. In this capacity the mediums are in competition with the male herbalists who have their own distinct view of illness. Among the most common complaints they hear are those related to childbearing and infertility. We will now look more closely at the different diagnoses and treatment dispensed by these two types of healers.

Today all the spirit mediums are women and the herbalists are men, although until about 15 years ago men, too, acted as mediums and the role of the head medium was always held by a man. Nowadays the mediums claim that it would be as difficult to persuade a man to become a medium as "to collect a pot of lice". This transition follows a pattern seen in other roles as well. Men receive the education which qualifies them for better jobs. They can, therefore, abandon some of their former positions in favour of those which bring them greater prestige and income. Women, who generally are not literate, have access to a comparatively narrower range of occupations but they now move into the positions which men have abandoned. It seems also that the restrictions imposed on the medium's personal life, as well as their official responsibilities, discourage men from taking up this profession today. Increasing numbers of men, however, are becoming herbalists. They too act as healers and have access to mystical power, with the important difference that they do not act as mediums of the spirits. In contrast to the roles of mediums which make rigorous demands on their personal lives, herbalists can practice their profession as it suits them. They are not under the authority of the Omanhene and are not obliged, as mediums are, to use their mystical powers to protect the community.

These two types of healers, the mediums and the herbalists, are not the only sources of mystical and medical aid available to the Aowins. There are also the Christian churches as well as the independent movements such as the Church of the Twelve Apostles, the government hospital and the Muslim healers. They have their respective techniques for treating problems of infertility. The hospital prescribes iron supplements and advises the woman to eat green vegetables while the independent churches use "holy water" to exorcise the evil spirit within her.

The Aowins rarely depend on just one healing specialist. If they do not meet with success at their first choice, they sample the remedies offered by another resource. An infertile woman may consult in succession all of the possibilities mentioned above. The order of succession, where she begins in her search for a cure, depends on the imprecise set of circumstances which shape any decision. Perhaps she has a kinsman who is active in the Methodist church or her brother obtained a job through the help of a herbalist. It is not possible to predict positively where she will go first but it is likely that if she does not meet with success she will continue to consult, in turn, all the specialists.

Fertility is a theme of crucial importance in the lives of the Aowin people. It is an index of the relationship of the Aowin state and the individual with the spirit world. The fertility of the land, the growth and abundance of the crops reflect the harmonious ties between the Aowin state and their gods. The invocations of the lineage heads, the Omanhene and spirit mediums are directed to ensure this fertility. The sterile man or woman is never fully accepted as a member of society. Barren women are suspected of being witches. Men who have no children are called derisive names and at the funeral of a childless person the corpse is abused as the mourners instruct the spirit of the dead person never to return again.

At the women's initiation rite, the *manzemua*, the concept of normal fertility is clearly defined. This rite is held after a girl has begun to menstruate and marks the commencement of her sexual life. In the past the rite lasted for three weeks but now it has been abbreviated to permit the girls to continue with their studies.

The rite is held in the compound of the girl's matrilineal kin. It is directed by a kinswoman who represents the Aowin model of motherhood. She has given birth to many children and her first-born child was a girl. This woman leads the girl, accompanied by her female kin and her friends, to the banks of the river where she is bathed. Her friends who have not yet begun to menstruate join her in this bath.

Women are credited with special mystical power which endows them with the ability to bear children, but this power, if not properly controlled, can transform the woman into a witch. Therefore all rituals and treatment related to childbearing focus on this "heat" of the woman which must be controlled for her own well-being and that of the community. Only after this instruction is it considered safe for the girl to conceive. Sexual intercourse before this time is seen as a grave misdemeanour (*monzue*), and a girl who becomes pregnant before the *manzemua* is harshly punished. In the past the child (*amu*) was killed at birth and even now such a child will not be allowed near the sacred areas. A girl who becomes pregnant with an *amu* child is sent to live in the forest until the birth and before she can return to the town she must pass through ritual purifications.

In initiation ceremonies the girl is ritually bathed, then rubbed with oil and dressed in a new cloth. The women dance and sing the *manzemua* songs as they lead her back to town. At the house where her friends have gathered, all share in a meal of *kokobekum*, a special dish of mashed yam and oil believed to make the girls fat and to make their skin shine. During the next two days, the girl and her friends are given rich stews of oil and meat. The senior woman feeds the *manzemua* girl and instructs her in the knowledge necessary to adult women. The old women also tell the girl how to care for her husband, to cook for him, to manage her household and to treat her husband and his kin with respect. Harmonious relations are believed to promote her fertility.

The rite transmits the knowledge she will need as a mother and it also establishes the model for her behaviour as a woman. The old women warn the girl that her behaviour during the *manzemua* will set the pattern for her future life. From this time onwards she should speak in a gentle voice and her movements should be dignified and quiet. Should she spill food on herself the old women shake their heads and predict that she will stain her clothes in that same spot every day for the rest of her life.

The rite presents a compressed view of a woman's life, from infancy to womanhood. On the first day, when she is carried to the river for the ritual bath, she is addressed as "infant". At the conclusion of the

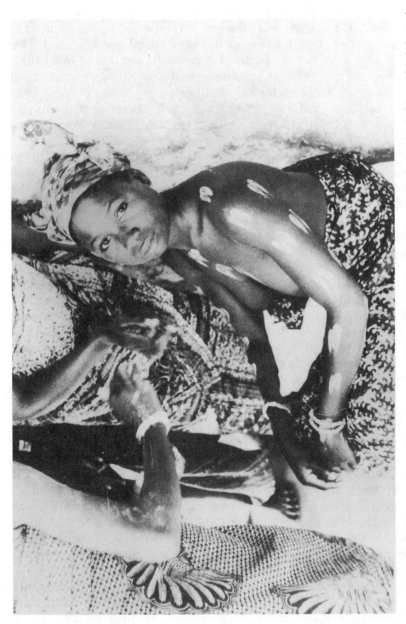

Fig. 2. As part of the women's initiation rite, the girl is painted with white clay, dressed in new clothes and led through the town.

manza week she is said to have become a woman (Rattray, 1927, p. 74). From now on she must abandon the play of her girlhood. The *manza* songs instruct her never to run in the streets again with the children and to spend her time with the women helping to prepare food and care for the children and the elderly. On the last day of the rite she is dressed in new clothes and the jewellery of her grandmother. She walks through the town, greeting the people who brought her gifts during the week, and on this final day, she is addressed by the term used for women who have just given birth.

By the performance of this rite, the Aowin people define their expectations of a woman's fertility. Let us now examine the recourses available to a woman when these expectations are not realized.

The Spirit Medium and Infertility

Each spirit medium has an appointed night during the week when she is consulted by clients. Among the group which gathers at her compound there are many women who are concerned because they are not yet pregnant. They describe their condition as *amoding* (literally "no name") a term which refers to a category of objects and states of being considered too dangerous to mention. To use the true name will evoke its evil presence into the everyday world. The initial task of the medium is to provide an interpretation of the affliction. Clearly, the gods or ancestors are angry with the woman, but what has she done to provoke their anger? As Horton notes (1967, p. 54) "the traditional diviner faced with a disease does not just refer to a spiritual agency. He uses ideas about this agency to link disease to causes in the world of visible tangible events". According to the mediums, the gods respond to the acts of individuals. The patient's social relationships are the central issue in the treatment. Misfortune is a consequence of troubled relations with the spirit world and it stems from the individual's acts which have generated the anger of the gods.

Over a period of several months, I collected the case histories of 25 women who attended the medium shrines with complaints of infertility. The mediums' diagnoses can be arranged in the following categories.

Witchcraft

Four women were told that witches had caused them to be infertile; one woman was told that she herself was a witch. Aowin descriptions of witches follow a pattern common throughout West Africa. McLeod in his discussion of Asante witches (1975, p. 11) notes that they represent an inversion of human traits and values. A witch goes naked through the night, sometimes flying upside down; she eats not with her mouth but with her anus, meeting her friends at night in the tall trees on the outskirts of the town. Barren women are frequently viewed as witches—they eat children instead of bearing them. The target of a witch's attack is her matrilineal kin, the focus of sentimental values and ties in this society. Jealousy is a key concept in the development of witchcraft powers. While anyone can be a witch, the individual who harbours jealousy is seen as most likely to become one. People are explicitly warned against envy for fear they will become witches. One is cautioned never to carry an object through the streets of the town without covering it from view lest anyone who catches sight of it should desire it and through envy bring misfortune to both bearer and observer.

In her diagnoses the medium draws attention to the tension which can arise within a matrilineal household. Women often remain with their matrilineal kin after they are married and here they are most exposed to the attacks of witches from among their own kin.

Non-observance of Prescribed Behaviour

Seven women were told they had offended the gods by not observing the traditional purificatory practices and by neglecting to give the gods the appropriate offerings. By this behaviour, the women had acquired pollution, *efeya*. The presence of *efeya* causes illness and is a particular threat to young children. An infant in close proximity with a menstruating woman, a potent source of pollution, may become ill because of her *efeya*. This same pollution can also prevent a woman from conceiving.

Disrupted Social Relationships

Nine women were told they would not conceive until they had reconciled their personal relationships. *Efeya* can also arise from animosity and feelings of ill will. A woman who quarrels with her neighbours, her co-wives or her husband will create a condition of pollution which causes her to become infertile. A woman's relationship with her husband is especially important.

When visiting a medium's shrine a woman usually comes alone or with her kinswomen, but those who complain of infertility are told they cannot be treated until they return with their husbands. The medium questions the woman closely, "Why has she neglected to inform him?", "Is she acting without his knowledge?", "Is he a devout Christian and therefore will he disapprove of the woman's presence at a medium's shrine?" or "Is the woman afraid that the medium will disclose that her promiscuous behaviour is the cause of her infertility?".

Quarrels between Matrilineal Kin

The bonds between matrilineal kin are a central focus in an individual's life. These ties order the rights to inheritance, the structure of household groups and are at the centre of an individual's affective relationships. A breach between matrilineal kin is considered a serious offence which creates a state of mystical danger known as *monzue*. It threatens the well-being of the community as well as the individuals whose offences have caused it to arise. Five women were told they were guilty of causing *monzue* because their behaviour had created tension within their matrilineal groups.

Treatment by the Mediums

In her treatment, the medium focusses on certain themes. These are (1) purification, (2) therapeutic remedies which also rely on the theme of purification, (3) reconciling social relations.

Purification

The infertile woman is said to be in a polluted state. She is described as "red" or "hot" and therefore dangerous. In the performance of the *momome*, the communal purificatory rite which centres around a ritual sweeping of the town, we can see that the spirit mediums are concerned with maintaining boundaries between the town and the forest, between "cool" and "hot". The town, a place of order, is defined against the unknown and dangerous properties of the forest. The presence of the infertile woman within the town violates this sense of order and she too is sent to the forest.

The forest is the source of mystical power and, therefore, it is a dangerous and unpredictable place. The river gods live there. Certain natural objects, *amoa*, treasured as magical charms, come from the forest. The *mmoatia*, the intermediaries between men and the forest also live there. They are described as small, red creatures who gave men their special knowledge of magical remedies and instructed them in how to make fire. There is also *Sasa Bonsam*, the forest monster described as enormously tall with long legs and flowing red hair. The objects and people associated with the forest and mystical power are also described as "red". The spirit mediums who acquire their special knowledge by spending long periods of time in the forest sing, "we are as red as possible". The Omanhene who needs mystical power to protect the Aowins from danger is called "Red Foot". Twins who by virtue of their birth are credited with special powers and are called "Men of the Forest" can be identified by their bracelets of red and white beads.

A bridge over the river marks the transition point between the forest and the town (McLeod, 1974). During the *momome* it is covered with white clay and becomes a barrier to keep spirits from the forest out of the town. To enter the town, objects and people associated with the red unpredictable power of the forest must be transformed; they must be made white and "cool". The shrine houses of the mediums, the Omanhene's palace, and the twins' households, are coated with white clay.

The transformation from red to white, from dangerous and hot to cool and safe, is a constant theme in the mediums' rites. At the beginning of each ritual performance, the mediums dress in the red cloth usually worn at funerals. Later, they exchange this for a white cloth with a red border; the completion of the rites is marked by the mediums' appearance in white. This theme is enacted throughout the performance. Red kola nuts coated with white clay are given as offerings to the gods. Eggs, which are an important element in the divinations, are smashed to the ground and the yolk, described as red, is immediately sprinkled with white clay.

Certain offences are also deemed as "red". A woman who becomes pregnant before she has passed through the *manzemua* has committed a "red" offence and she is sent to live in the forest. Serious crimes, such as murder, incest, and giving birth to a tenth child, are also classified as "red" and the mediums must rid the community of this danger. In the past, the individual may have been killed. Now he or she is banished to the forest and led through purificatory rites. The infertile woman is also described as dangerous, "hot" and "red". For her too the forest is the appropriate place until she has been purified.

This purification can take different forms. The woman who has acquired *efeya* by neglecting to give offerings to the god or by quarrelling with a non-kinsman is bathed in the river and gives a modest offering such as a hen and eggs to the gods. Afterwards the medium paints the woman with white clay, dresses her in white cloth and leads her

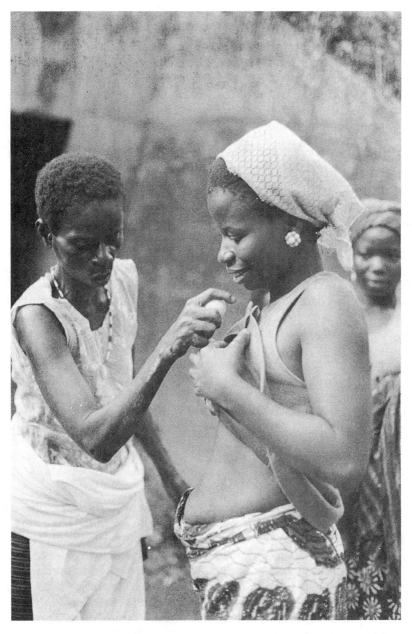

Fig. 3. A priestess passes an egg over the belly of a pregnant woman which is said to cleanse her of harmful pollution. Afterwards, the egg is smashed to the ground and the priestess claims to be able to divine the state of the woman's pregnancy.

back to town. For more serious offences, those which threaten the safety of the town, the rites become more elaborate. The woman spends a few weeks with the medium at her shrine in the forest where she is given daily remedies valued for their cleansing properties. For example, she can eat only foods described as white and she bathes everyday in a mixture of water from a sacred river, white clay and leaves. At the end of this period, on an appointed day, her kinsmen come to the shrine in the forest and through the medium, she gives an offering of a sheep to appease the gods and asks them to remove the *monzue*.

Medical Treatment Provided by the Spirit Mediums

The mediums also rely on herbal and arboreal remedies but they admit that many of these are common-place and can be easily obtained. They describe these remedies in terms of their purifying qualities and their effectiveness in eliminating the pollution. They stress the cleansing, whitening action of certain compounds. Each medium counts among her valued remedies the roots of a certain plant which are white and shiny. Powdered white clay is added to most mixtures especially those which are to be used as a douche. The medium also relies on purgatives to help infertile women; they give mixtures to use as enemas which contain pepper, ginger and other harsh substances. To treat some cases, the medium applies a cupping horn to the abdomen to extract the "bad blood" *mogya feya* from the body.

Despite the simple nature of their remedies, people still continue to consult the mediums. While their medicines can be easily obtained elsewhere, only the mediums can perform the purificatory rites, and for these, the Aowin are content to pay.

Reconciling Social Relations

The spirit mediums, in their interpretation of misfortune, emphasize harmonious social relationships. The tension and hostility between two individuals can threaten the well-being of the entire community. Often the mediums will act as informal adjudicators and will intervene to give their opinions in cases of dispute. For a woman who is infertile, her social relationships are a central issue in the diagnosis of her complaint. She must reconcile her relationships with her kin and neighbours as well as her husband. The medium organizes the reconciliation and calls upon them to attend this final stage of the woman's treatment. After the purification has been performed and the woman is dressed in white they all share in a ceremonial meal.

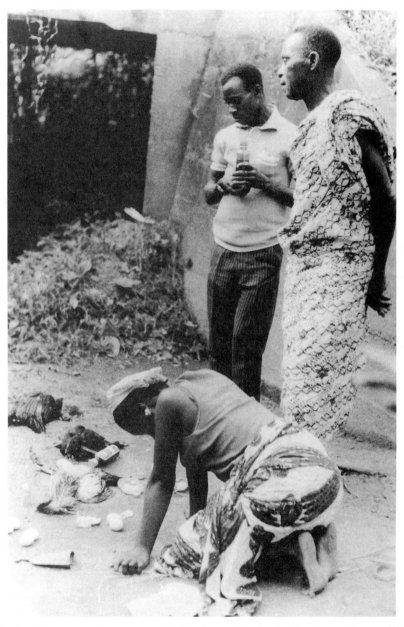

Fig. 4. A woman makes offerings to the river god and asks him to grant her a child.

The medium also takes on the responsibility for reconciling disputes on the spirit level. When a woman is infertile due to witchcraft the medium undertakes to appease the witch. The central point mentioned above in the description of the witch is that she is jealous. By offering gifts to the witch, as the medium claims to do at night, her ravenous spirit is appeased.

The medium's treatment is directed towards maintaining the fabric of social life. As an office-holder in the Omanhene's court she has a responsibility to maintain good relations between his subjects. In her view of the world, good health depends on good behaviour. She attempts to regulate the quality of life within the town; she urges good social relations and cohesive kin ties and upholds a certain order in community life which is manifested in the use of space and in maintaining the boundaries between states of purity and pollution.

Let us now compare this view of infertility with its emphasis on stable social and kin relationships and the observance of communal rules with the interpretation of infertility dispensed by the herbalists.

The Herbalists

In Enchi, there are nine men who practise as herbalists. Unlike the mediums they are not part of the political hierarchy and are not under the jurisdiction of a superior. While the mediums emphasize the conservative values associated with political authority and the traditional standards of behaviour, the herbalists make use of their Western education and exposure to Western ways. Some are well educated by Enchi standards and they all speak English; one is a school-teacher. On the whole, these men are a prosperous group: they are cocoa farmers, mechanics and craftsmen. For all these men Western thought has played some part in their healing techniques and they augment their traditional remedies with the terms and concepts they have learned from school science books.

Diagnosis and Treatment Provided by the Herbalist

The herbalist also receives clients at the shrines of his tutelary spirits. He too gives offerings to these spirits who in exchange help him to heal. While he depends on them as the medium does, he can also draw upon the extensive knowledge of herbal and arboreal remedies he acquired during his apprenticeship. The medium too must pass through

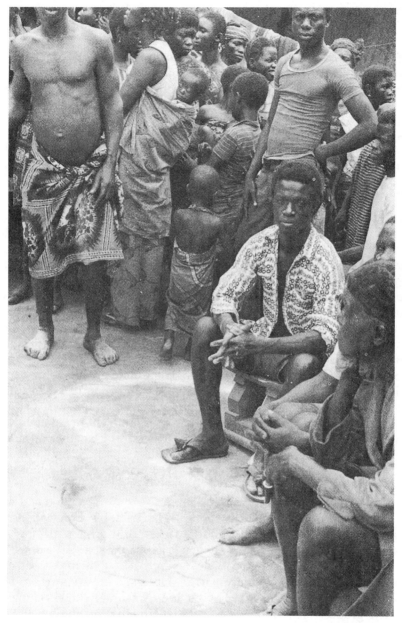

Fig. 5. A herbalist is accused of sabotaging the priestesses' efforts to "call the gods".
He is brought forward and a circle of white clay is drawn around him which is said
to limit his nefarious activities.

an apprenticeship but this time is devoted to adapting to a new way of life, learning how to enter into trances, to dance for the gods, to conduct rites. The herbalist has spent his time learning the properties of leaves and the appropriate remedies for specific afflictions. Even after the apprenticeship has ended he continues to learn new remedies. The herbalists trade such knowledge with each other and sometimes travel great distances, to Upper Volta and to Ivory Coast, to acquire new and, they hope, more powerful healing remedies and charms with magical powers. The acquisition of this sort of knowledge is essential to attracting new clients and forms the basis of a herbalist's prestige. The herbalists energetically collect new formulas and recipes which are quickly discarded in favour of new and more sensational cures.

In his treatment of illness the herbalist relies on the knowledge he has acquired. His techniques are based on the patient's physical symptoms. While the medium immediately looks for an explanation of affliction in the woman's social relationships, the herbalist offers an explanation based on an anatomical model of the processes necessary for conception. Some of the herbalists use their interest in lorry engines to explain the dynamics of human physiology. They compare the human body to a lorry engine with its intermeshed gears and power-charged batteries. Madness, for example, is caused when two parallel "wires" in the temple are brought into contact with the brain, resulting in sparks and explosions. The herbalists base their explanation for many sorts of dysfunctions on this model. For example, impotence is explained by this analogy. They claim that a wire connects a man's nose to his penis and, as his heart beats quickly in passion, the wire tightens and causes him to ejaculate. A man becomes impotent in old age when the string becomes lax or when he is "cursed" by another, a fate to which an adulterer is particularly susceptible. The herbalist gives this explanation to his client as he administers the remedy to restore the connecting wire to its former tautness.

The herbalist can also explain certain facts about conception and how a child comes to resemble his father. He bases his explanations on traditional beliefs about the *ntoro*, the patrilineal transmitted "soul" or "spirit". Rattray (1923, p. 46) defines it as, "That spiritual element in a man or a woman, upon which depends . . . that force, personal magnetism, character, worldly power, success in any venture, in fact, everything which makes life worth living". Each individual belongs to a *ntoro* group which, in the past, met regularly to give offerings to their common spirit. From his mother the individual inherited *mogya*, the blood, which determines his allegiance to a matrilineal group. The combination of these two elements composes the individual but they do not always mix harmoniously. Sometimes, a woman explains that she cannot conceive because her *mogya* does not mix well with the *ntoro* of her husband.

While a woman is pregnant she must observe the taboos demanded by her husband's spirit or she may miscarry. Adultery is a grave offence for a pregnant woman because it brings two *ntoro* spirits into conflict. The herbalist claims to be able to see *ntoro* and explain its role in the physiology of sex and conception. He explains that as a man ejaculates, all thoughts are driven from his head, his mind is empty. The herbalist takes this explanation as literally true and describes the white waxy substance in the brain which shoots down to a man's penis.

To explain conception to his patients, the herbalist describes the rotating action of the womb which he compares to a gear shift. Its revolution is on a 30-day cycle which explains the regularity of menstruation. The womb is said to be composed of small compartments, and it is in one of these that the foetus develops. According to this model, at some time in the woman's life, an accumulation of *efeya* may cause the gear shift to stop. They say this occurs because the woman has not taken the ritual bath which is prescribed after intercourse and at the end of the menstrual cycle. This blockage prevents conception and also provides an explanation for the menopause.

During the consultation the herbalist asks his client questions which are related to his model of the human body. "How often does the woman menstruate?" "Does she have frequent intercourse?" The herbalist formulates his treatment according to her response. One woman who complained of aches and pains all over her body was told her blood was so thick that it coursed sluggishly and caused her pain. She could not conceive because her blood was too heavy to mix with the semen. This malady had developed because she ate too much cassava, described as slimy and heavy. To correct her condition he gave her some leaves to thin out the blood. The medium confronted with a similar case of a man who had swellings under his skin was told that the lump was caused by *efeya* which arose because of his surly attitude to his wife.

The treatment of the herbalist is directed to the patient's complaint. He is not interested in her personal relationships, either with the community or with the spirit world. Her behaviour does not affect her state of health and to this healer she does not have to explain her conduct. The herbalist's focus on the physical aspects of her affliction represents a departure from the world view of the medium.

Conclusion

We have looked at the contrasting views of fertility held by men and women healers in this society. For the mediums, infertility is not seen merely as an individual malady but it becomes the focal point from which to view the client's relationship with the social universe. A case of infertility reflects a disturbance in the community; it is an index of the quality of social relations and relations between men and the gods. The medium's interpretation of infertility pin-points areas of tension in the town and, as an official of the Omanhene's court, she has a responsibility to correct this situation. She attempts to maintain order in social relationships and to ensure a harmonious relationship between humans and the spirit world.

The medium represents the conservative elements in Aowin life to-day. She upholds traditional values, promotes stable marriages and relations between kin. In her view the community is a defined unit, bound together by ties of kinship and mutual obligation. In her rites she illustrates her view of spatial relations between the town and the forest. She outlines the town in white against the dangers and chaos of the forest. From her point of view an infertile woman represents an element of disorder which allies her with the mystical power associated with the forest. Disorders related to childbearing and fertility are highly threatening to the community; they are a violation of the order which separates the social universe from the spirit world. The medium's treatment revolves around the transformation of the opposed concepts of dangerous and safe, heat and cool, polluted and pure. These themes are conceptualized during the treatment in the use of space between the forest and the town and in the use of red and white. As a healer, under the authority of the Omanhene, the medium is concerned not only with the individual client but with the well-being of the community as a whole. In her view of the world, every member of the society is a catalyst to which others are vulnerable. She treats the infertile woman and at the same time protects the community from the harm she may bring.

The herbalists represent a different point of view. They have always differed from the mediums in that they acquire their capacity to heal by learning while the mediums heal through their association with the spirits, by direct inspiration from the gods. The medium's period of apprenticeship concentrates on affirming her relationship with the spirits while the herbalist spends his time learning remedies. Moreover, today the herbalists are men who have been exposed to Western values and education. For them, the emphasis is on the individual, not on his or her social relationships. The concept of the community is not relevant to his view of illness. For him there is no need to look beyond the individual to discover an explanation of his problems. The medium, on the other hand, wants to control and regulate childbearing. A woman should conceive only after the *manzemua* has been performed, in the order of birth only certain children are acceptable, intercourse is approved only with certain people and within the limits of the town. Sexuality and childbearing are brought within the domain of culture and are integrated into an overall view of the social universe. To the herbalist, with his emphasis on learning and models of the workings of the body, childbearing is not part of an overall world view. To him it is a different sort of problem, one which can be seen as a discrete and isolated occurrence and not one which reflects the core of man's relationships with the social and mystical worlds.

References

Busia, K. A. (1954). "The Ashanti of the Gold Coast". In *African Worlds: Studies in Cosmological Ideas and Social Values of African Peoples* (D. Forde, ed.). Oxford: Oxford University Press.

Fortes, M. (1950). "Kinship and Marriage Among the Ashanti". In *African Systems of Kinship and Marriage* (A. R. Radcliffe-Brown and D. Forde, eds). Oxford: Oxford University Press.

Fortes, M. (1969). *Kinship and the Social Order*. London: Routledge and Kegan Paul.

Fortes, M. (1970). *Time and Social Structure and Other Essays*. New York: Humanities Press.

Goody, E. (1973). *Contexts of Kinship: an Essay in the Family Sociology of the Gonja of Northern Ghana*. Cambridge: Cambridge University Press.

Horton, R. (1967). "African Traditional Thought and Western Science". *Africa* **37**, 50–71.

Hubert, H. and Mauss, M. (1964). *Sacrifice: Its Nature and Function*. Chicago: University of Chicago Press.

McLeod, M. (1974). Exhibition of Asante. Unpublished manuscript. Haddon Museum, Cambridge.

McLeod, M. (1975). "On the Spread of Anti-witchcraft Cults in Modern Asante". In *Changing Social Structure in Ghana* (J. Goody, ed.). London: International African Institute.

Rattray, R. S. (1923). *Ashanti*. Oxford: Clarendon Press.

Rattray, R. S. (1927). *Religion and Art in Ashanti*. Oxford: Clarendon Press.

Rattray, R. S. (1929). *Ashanti Law and Constitution*. Oxford: Oxford University Press.

6. Folk Medicine and Fertility: Aspects of Yoruba Medical Practice Affecting Women

U. MACLEAN

The activities of various categories of Yoruba healers have received increasing attention, ever since the late 1950s (Rudolph, 1965; Jahn, 1962; Parrinder, 1953; Idowu, 1962; Lambo, 1964). Lately the World Health Organization has stimulated interest in those forms of medicine which are generally the sole resort of the great mass of the population in developing countries, far from urban centres and the possibility of high powered modern therapeutic intervention (WHO, 1978).

From the anthropological point of view, Lloyd (1967) has made a brief reference to Yoruba medical practitioners, whilst Little (1966) mentioned the importance in West Africa today of voluntary organizations, to which many herbalists belong. Verger (1957, 1966), whose main interest has been the persistent links between Yoruba culture and its survivals in contemporary Brazil, has contributed notably to the subject, not only by his massive work on the *orisha* (gods) including those specifically connected with illness, but also by his interest in the praise names (*oriki*) of various medicinal plants and on the use of tranquilizers and stimulants in the Yoruba pharmacopoeia.

What might be termed the general, day-to-day practice of these Yoruba healers has been mentioned by Ajose (1957) and also by several Ibadan medical students in a little known clinical journal (Atalabi, 1964). But there is no special attention given to women's needs or to women practitioners.

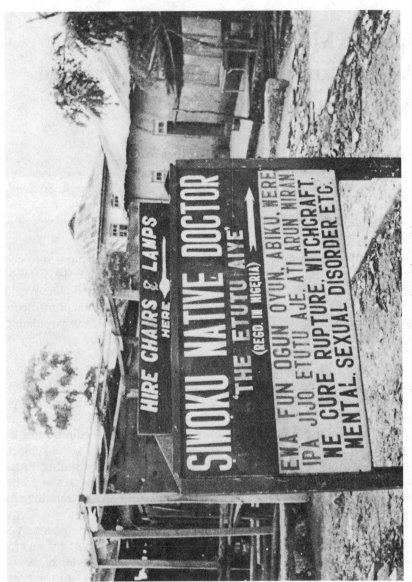

Fig. 1.   Yoruba traditional practitioner.

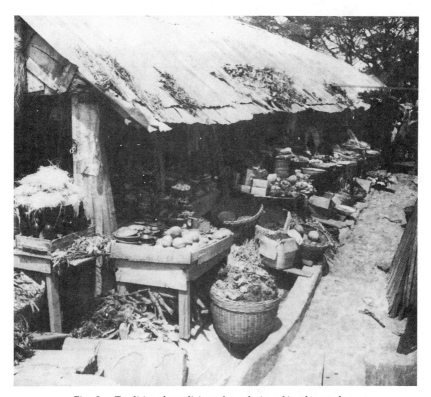

Fig. 2. Traditional medicines for sale in a Yoruba market.

In other publications I have described the African healers practising in the city of Ibadan (Maclean, 1965, 1966, 1969, 1971).

Yoruba traditional practitioners are still very much in evidence. They fall into two main groups, herbalists and diviners. The Onishegun or herbalist will have learned about a very large number of herbal preparations since first being apprenticed as a young boy in the service of a senior healer. Herbalists not only recognize the pharmacological properties of different plants and their use in day-to-day medical practice but are concerned with making them up as ointments, soaps, embroications and solutions of various kinds. Some of the medicines in common use do have a direct biochemical action within the body when absorbed, but in many other cases the effectiveness of a remedy depends on principles of sympathetic magic, deriving from a symbolic resemblance between one or other of the ingredients and the condition for which they are prescribed.

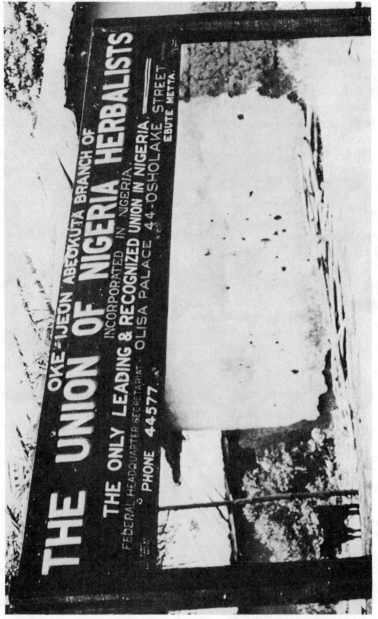

Fig. 3.   Union of herbalists.

During the collection of plants from the bush special praise songs or *oriki* are sung, which make explicit their desired medicinal power. When a magical remedy is being employed an incantation is again necessary, to incorporate the influence of the spoken human word, without which matter alone is neutral and negligible.

There is in the herbalist's materia medica a division between simple medicaments which are prepared for imbibing or for applying to the body externally to relieve common physical symptoms and those which are intended to operate at a distance. These are really charms and countercharms and have nothing to do with the modern science of pharmacology. Some of them are intended to produce a beneficial or satisfactory effect on the patient himself or on someone close to him. Others are aimed at modifying the behaviour of influential outsiders. Others may be necessary to counteract the suspected malevolence of enemies. Then there are talismans to promote good fortune and protect the wearer from general or specific dangers. The latter are essentially prophylactic, taken today to ensure a healthy and prosperous tomorrow. All of these require that the user should have faith in their efficacy. Ideally the healer too should believe in his own medicines and should not be a mere charlatan or quack, falsely advertizing the virtues of remedies he knows to be worthless.

Much of the herbalist's regular trade is concerned with the provision of medicines for simple ailments, but they sometimes employ a form of divination in difficult cases which are not responding to treatment.

For expertise in diagnosis by divination, however, someone in serious, persistent trouble will consult a *Babalawo*, one of the priests of *Ifa* (fate). They are able to uncover deeper causes of disease or misfortune than are within the capacity of the ordinary Onishegun. They employ a complicated system, involving the repeated casting of 16 kola nuts from one hand to the other. All the results, in terms of odd or even numbers, are recorded on a sanded tray and then referred to the diviner's memory of 256 verses or sayings in the *Odu* or corpus of knowledge of the Ifa cult. When recited to the anxious supplicant the verses which have been turned up by this chance process will convey a special significance which can be interpreted as a message fitted to his or her own circumstances. Fate, once revealed, then proves to be capable of manipulation by suitable, wise action or precautions.

The divination process as practised by the Yoruba *babalawo* does not involve trance but is frequently accompanied by elaborate ritual sacrifice. Any exchange between the patient and his or her spiritual adviser relates to personal relationships or to the observance or neglect of religious observances and is far removed from the concentration upon physical symptoms of most modern, medical diagnosticians. It is best to regard the *babalawo* as psychotherapists who are concerned with the web of social relationships surrounding a patient and affecting his or her sense of well-being and control over events.

The two main categories of indigenous, Yoruba healers are supplemented by Hausa barber surgeons and sellers of Moslem remedies, bone setters, circumcisers and, in growing numbers, prophets of several Apostolic Churches. The latter churches combine features of Christianity and paganism and their charismatic healers have a reputation for dealing with psychiatric patients.

Yoruba herbalists are becoming a pressure group for official recognition. They have long been in the habit of forming professional associations to protect their interests. In the present climate of opinion, with even the prestigious World Health Organization calling for the promotion of traditional therapies, they feel more confident and are very unlikely to agree to surveillance by doctors from the rival Western system.

Early in my investigations in Nigeria I was concentrating upon the continued use of folk remedies by two contrasting sections of the population; on the one hand the inhabitants of an old quarter of the town, very like a village, consisting mainly of traditional type housing and on the other those élite families who could afford secondary education for their children.

The research was prompted by the need to discover the relationship of age and sex to the utilization of modern medical facilities and was incidental to an epidemiological study of the incidence rates of different cancers in a defined population. Because the crude rate of cancer among the older sections of the population turned out to be low when compared with American or European figures, a sociological study was undertaken among these contrasting groups of the city's inhabitants to discover their views upon the efficacy of hospitals as a source of help with various illnesses. As the results were analysed the important influence which women were having upon their families' usage of hospitals as opposed to traditional treatments became apparent.

Almost 60% of families at either end of the social scale were occasionally employing local treatment methods but mothers who had received some training for a profession, such as teaching or nursing, positively discouraged the use of traditional medicines in their households. On the other hand, uneducated young mothers were already developing the habit of taking their small infants to hospital when their illness was serious, even if it meant defying the older men in the family compound whose prerogative it had always formerly been to decide upon such action.

West African societies still experience extremely high rates of infant mortality. The anticipation of child loss has been paralleled by deep concern for the perpetuation of the family. This has been remarked on by Lambo (1956), referring to women presenting themselves at psychiatric clinics with secondary, psychosomatic symptoms due to their failure to conceive. The same has frequently been noted by practising obstetricians (Lawson, 1967).

The life of the barren woman is undoubtedly a miserable one; she may easily be displaced to make room for a fertile wife; she is denied the pleasures and pre-occupation of child rearing; in later life she is without the support of sons and daughters, upon whose work and affectionate attention she might otherwise have hoped to depend.

The Yoruba woman is not merely concerned with her capacity to conceive and bear children but also with ensuring their survival through the highly perilous months and years of infancy. It is still possible for all of a woman's children to die before reaching five years of age. Thus, even the most fertile woman can be ultimately left childless, rendering the continuation of her husband's descent line dependent upon rival wives in a polygamous household.

For a more intensive investigation of women's continued reliance upon traditional healers and practices, interviews were carried out with women from a one in five sample of households in the same Ibadan ward which had featured in the previous survey and with a similar sized group of women from Idere, a rural village 50 miles to the north-west. They were questioned about beliefs and practices relating to pregnancy, labour and infant care. Special reference was made to the possible use of local medicines during these stages and to consultations with traditional practitioners. They were asked about the utilization of hospitals or clinics and for their views on the management of some common childhood ailments. At the same time a subsidiary enquiry was carried out among 100 Ibadan herbalists, focussing attention on the extent and nature of their treatment of women's and children's complaints (Maclean, 1969). Locally printed pamphlets were also studied.

The women in the large city of Ibadan had relatively easy access to several hospitals with up-to-date maternity facilities. The village women, on the other hand, could make use of a small, four-bedded, maternity unit in the neighbouring small town of Igbo-Ora, five miles away. A health centre has been established here, primarily as a site for teaching medical students. The resources for care are strictly limited and midwifery is in the hands of one nursing sister who can only occasionally depend on a doctor being available. Difficult cases have to be transferred by local transport to the distant city.

Almost the same number of interviews were carried out in Ibadan (99) and in Idere village (108). The majority of the women whom the student interviewers approached were co-operative, but sometimes an explanation of the purpose of the enquiry had to be provided by a senior Yoruba medical attendant. On other occasions, women might refuse to take part without their husband's consent, but this was usually easily obtained. Some elderly women could not believe that anyone should want to hear their opinion, but other old women were flattered by such attention and wanted to talk at great length and not always precisely to the point.

It had to be accepted that interviews could not possibly be a private affair between the interviewer and the respondent. In West Africa the whole family expect to join in answering a questionnaire, prompting the central person, aiding her memory, correcting her mistakes and arguing over points of detail.

Asked about their use of folk remedies for treating childrens' ailments, the village women all reported that they had used them. But amongst the younger women in the Ibadan group the use of such medicines was less general. There were similar contrasts between town and village in relation to the women's choice of different facilities during confinement. Although village women could, if they so desired, attend the Igbo-Ora Health Centre to give birth, few of the patients there had come from Idere (Barber, 1966). In response to questions about their experience of hospital or health centre, 30% of Ibadan women reported having given birth in hospital, whilst only 14% of Idere women had delivered in the local unit. Possibly the facilities there are insufficient to attract women from the comforting and familiar security of their own homes.

As far as the use of traditional medicines during labour at home was concerned, again this was much more common amongst village women. But both town and country mothers had used traditional medicines and consulted traditional practitioners to the same extent regarding the means of ensuring conception and of avoiding infertility. In this intimate area of their lives none of them anticipated much success from the unaided efforts of European trained doctors. They preferred to trust in established magical medicines, rituals and routines recommended by herbalists and diviners for generations.

The interviews uncovered details regarding the local management of pregnancy and labour. The husband is responsible for obtaining certain medicines which he may consider necessary for his wife's successful pregnancy. Thus he may obtain the materials to construct a protective charm or see to it that his wife regularly drinks an infusion, or herbal soup, containing specific plants which are highly regarded by local herbalists.[1]

The large, African variety of snail should form an important part of the diet of expectant mothers; similarly, pregnant women are encouraged to eat mice and tortoises. These foods are in no way exotic or unusual, in fact they constitute valuable sources of dietary protein in a region where all large game has by now been exterminated and where dried fish or fresh beef are much too expensive for most people's regular use.

Pregnant women are, however, warned against eating large plaintains whose longitudinal cleft is believed to promote a tendency to difficult labour, followed by the birth of a child with a "ridged" skull. This may refer to the rare condition of hydrocephalus. More probably it simply reflects the common pre-occupation of mothers in many cultures with the state of their infant's fontanelles.

A woman in this condition ought to avoid work by a roadside, the well known route of evil influences and the favoured position for the planting of evil spells. When sitting down, the pregnant woman should see that no one steps over her outstretched legs, for fear they may bequeath their likeness to her unborn child.

There is no special class of traditional midwives to assist the Yoruba woman in labour. She kneels or squats upon the floor, alone in a room by herself during the first stage. However, later on, assistance may be provided by an elderly female relative, who has the benefit of personal experience and attendance at numerous other deliveries. The herbalist or diviner may be summoned to prescribe remedies and procedures in cases of special difficulty. Vaginal examination or interference does not take place, though external abdominal pressure may be employed.

Informants from both town and village referred to certain specific herbal mixtures in current use. Intra-abdominal pressure is sometimes raised when the stage of expelling the placenta is reached by thrusting a wooden pastle down the woman's throat, causing her to gag or vomit.

After birth the child's cord is cut with any handy sharp instrument, a sliver of bamboo, a piece of broken glass, a knife or razor blade. A bath is then given, using local "black" soap and a fibre sponge and the next oldest child may be given the bath water to drink, possibly to convey new vigour to him. A piece of heated stone or potshead wrapped in wet cloth is applied to the umbilicus. The ashes from the parents' burnt sleeping mat are used as dressing.[2] The afterbirth is taken and buried outside the house, close by the side of the dwelling.

Small drinks of weak corn flour paste are offered first since breast milk is not considered suitable when it is in its early form. Breast-feeding does not begin until two or three days after birth. There is clearly a high risk of contamination at this stage of artificial feeding. The child may continue to have drinks at the breast for anything up to four years. Being favoured above girls, boys are breast-fed, on average, for longer than their sisters. Formerly, the spacing of births was ensured by a contraceptive rule which prohibited intercourse whilst breast-feeding continued but, partly because of the decline in polygamy, the rule is now less universally observed. However, the women respondents insisted that a pregnancy arising during lactation would be likely to prove injurious to both the suckling child and to the one newly conceived.[3] Final weaning is often established by applying to the nipple bitter substances which will discourage sucking.

Many women, in both Ibadan and Idere, were firmly convinced that an older woman who had herself borne children could undertake the suckling of an infant whose mother had died. The local use of a herbal mixture might, they said, be necessary to induce lactation in such cases. The women had observed that this phenomenon was more common formerly than nowadays, when the availability of tinned and dried milks lessened the immediate crisis for an orphaned child. However, supplementary or artificial feeding with proprietary dried or condensed milk later on is very dangerous indeed when prepared in the unhygienic circumstances most women have to endure (Jelliffe and Jelliffe, 1977). Moreover, the mixture is seldom made up to proper strength. Without a register of births and deaths maintained for a period of years it is impossible to balance the past and present risks to village women's children and the resultant change in total numbers of survivors.

One of the spiritual dangers lying in wait for pregnant women are thought to be the spirits of *abiku* who may try to usurp the child in her womb if she is foolish enough to go out at night.

Abiku children are "born to die"; after living with their parents for only a little while, they leave to rejoin their spirit companions who have always been tempting them to return. Sometimes, it is believed, the same *abiku* child will come back time and again to torment the parents with its temporary presence, only to die in due course. A pregnant woman will try to avoid the attentions of *abiku* by tying a knot in her wrapper if she cannot avoid a night journey. And once an *abiku* child is born to her, if she suspects its true nature, she can call it special names, pathetically urging it to stay like, "Sit down and play with me", or "Remain to bury me". She may pamper and indulge it, giving in to its every whim, hoping against hope that she may succeed in making its mortal home too attractive to leave.

The *abiku* child which has returned a second or subsequent time can, it is thought, be recognized by some distinctive feature of mark. Unlike their stronger companions, children thought to be *abiku* are not circumcised in infancy. The operation may be delayed until they are old enough to marry, by which time their survival has been assured.

This belief in *abiku* children may be operating as a necessary and ingenious explanation for the high rate of infant deaths, providing a satisfactory framework within which such distressing episodes may be accepted.

It is worth noting in passing how small infants, in Yoruba traditional culture as in many others, are not regarded as possessing full individuality. They are looked upon as an appurtenance of their mother until at least the age of seven years. Infant deaths are not the occasion of general adult mourning; the mother bewails, in wild, abandoned weeping, their untimely demise, which is less noisily grieved by the males in the family.

Seven Idere women and five Ibadan women mentioned local deities whom they served. This was in spite of the modern tendency to conceal personal adherence to pagan gods and cults and to claim connections with the more reputable Moslem or Christian faiths. The god, *Ogun* is believed to be particularly favourable towards appeals for offspring. Although he is primarily the god of war and of all dealers in iron, his powers extend in other directions as well. The faith of one *Ogun* worshipper remained unshaken although she had lost all her eight children in early infancy.

The beautiful river god, *Yemaja*, requires of her worshippers that they come silently to the riverbank for water each morning and return without greeting anyone. The children of *Yemaja* should have cowrie shells placed in their drinking and bathing water.

The Yoruba have the highest rate of twin births in the world (55 per 1000) and special ceremonies follow their birth. The first born of twins or *Ibeji* is named *Taiwo* and the second is *Kehinde*. The usual rejoicing over a single birth are multiplied in this lucky event and the mother is showered with gifts and blessings. Later she is expected to dance in the streets and receive offerings on their behalf. The former custom of having small carvings to represent twins is now, unfortunately, almost lost. Previously, if a twin died, a specially commissioned carving was placed in the family shrine and tended with great care.[4] Sometimes the doll-like figure was carried around by the surviving twin. The *Ibeji* carvings seen in Idere in 1965 were most inferior, some consisting merely of a roughly shaped cylinder of wood in marked contrast to those made by an earlier generation of skilled craftsmen and still to be found in many public and private collections.

The Hundred Healers

These healers were identified by hearsay and were interviewed with the help of a Yoruba research assistant. They all proved very co-operative and, whilst they were grateful for the small financial token of appreciation which was given at the close of an interview, they did not demand remuneration beforehand.

Thirty-seven of those interviewed referred to themselves as *onishegun* (herbalists), 60 were diviner priests of Ifa (*babalawo*), there was one faith healer and two who did not specify the main nature of their practice. Two of the healers were women. Two-thirds of them were over 45 years of age and 20 were over 65.

Twenty stated they had been taught by their fathers, eight by another member of the family. The remainder had been apprenticed to specialists, many of whom practised outside the city of Ibadan. The period of apprenticeship varied, but it averaged eight or nine years, although some had studied for over 15 years and six declared that they were still learning. In 27 cases the healing art had been a family speciality and 20 of them reported that there had also been women healers among their relatives. Whilst there were five who restricted their practice to women's ailments the remainder maintained that they could cure all or most diseases.

Almost all of them were in the habit of prescribing for women in labour and 98 considered themselves competent to deal with convulsions in children. Twenty-three of them detailed a particular recipe for the medicine which they used for this symptom.

Fifty-eight said that they were able to treat "diseases due to witchcraft" and 43 specified an actual anti-witchcraft remedy.

Questioned about the use of a number of particular herbal remedies, they repeatedly referred to a variety of plants specifically intended to ensure conception, to help pregnant women, to relieve menstrual irregularities and to treat childrens' ailments. (The details of these are to be reported elsewhere.)

Two Ibadan Practitioners

The circumstances of actual practitioners can be well conveyed by two descriptive illustrations. Mr. S.A. was interviewed in his home in a traditional quarter of the town. He was a spare, fine-featured man in his forties. He ushered the visitors into his room in the compound and prepared to demonstrate some of his procedures.

The room was dark and dingy; in the space below the foot of the bed and the wall, black pots of various sizes were grouped and, beneath the bed, in bottles, were herbs and roots. A group of four small indifferently carved *Ibeji* (twin cult) figures stood with scraps of palm oil paste placed as an offering before them. Hung about the walls were bunches of feathers and indeterminate medicines as charms. In one corner near the bed, in a slight of white cloth, a bunch of dried grasses of light yellowish colour lit up the gloom. This, it transpired, was a powerful counter-charm against witchcraft.

Mr. A. had learnt his trade from his father. In his family there were no women with knowledge of local medicine. He declared that his most popular medicines were those to ensure conception. A group of herbs in a small gourd were pointed out as the constituents of one such mixture, they were eventually to be dissolved in lime juice. Mr. A. asserted that his purges, tonics and mixtures for barren women obviated the need for surgical intervention.

Mr. A. also claimed that he was able to induce lactation in post-menopausal women by the use of a medicine applied to the breast. These would be effective within two or three days. He seemed surprised to hear that this skill was unknown in Europe or America.

Medicines for children were in constant demand. A mother called during my visit and was told to return with an empty bottle. Although it appeared initially as though he only used direct diagnosis and no divination it had, however, been observed that among the objects in his room was a small Ifa board with a little yellow powder on it. He showed how he made certain marks on it with two fingers. It appeared that divination did form an important aspect of his primarily herbal craft.

About most of his business there seemed to be nothing secret. But he maintained that the preparation of certain medicines had to be attended with great secrecy and was much too dangerous for women to witness since to do so might render them barren. He himself personally knew certain women who had deserved reputations as diviners.

Mr. R.A.R. was an elderly Ibadan man who came somewhat reluctantly for interview at the University. He recalled how, by the time he was eight, he began to accompany his father to gather herbs in the forest and used to pay careful attention to the advice which his father gave to suppliants. After a prolonged apprenticeship, he was able, by the age of 25, to set up on his own. At the time of the interview, he himself was employing several apprentices. He had learnt certain elements of his skill from his mother. Although her type of medicine involved less ceremony, her knowledge was unquestionable. "Women are witches", was his own explanation for the particular potency of his mother's remedies.

He declared that he personally knew of cases of old women who had been able to breast-feed children following upon the local application of some medicine. A liquid preparation also had to be taken by mouth to induce lactation and the effect of the drugs would be obvious within 24 hours.

Yoruba Medical Books

In the course of my enquiries into different aspects of Yoruba medicine I discovered booklets written in Yoruba and locally printed for sale in the local market, containing assorted recipes or prescriptions for local medicines. The public for such pamphlets would presumably have to be persons who had learnt to read Yoruba at school—clerks, technicians and so on whom one might have expected to be losing touch with these aspects of their culture.

When translated, the material which came to light is of great interest for the light which casts upon the Yoruba concept of medicine. The passages quoted make it abundantly clear that medicines are not seen to depend for their effect solely upon the pharmacological potency of the drugs which they contain.

The first booklet goes by the title of *"Awakaiye"*, which is roughly translatable as, The Fruit of Universal Knowledge. The introduction begins with a song of praise or *Oriki*: "Words of Reverence". Next follow some Words of Advice, which clearly indicate the talismanic purpose of much of its contents. "We have written this book for the use of all the Yoruba people, for curing them and for protecting them from the wrath and machinations of wicked people".

Among prophylactics against impotence, curses for gonorrhoea, recipes for luck and energy and foresight is the following remedy. "To prevent miscarriage: One tortoise to be cooked in coconut milk mixed with half a bottle of palm oil. Allow it to boil until all the liquid has been driven off and then grind up the meat. Some of it should be mixed in *eko* (a cornflour pudding). The woman should take it in the morning and at night, from the time when she begins menstruating until she finishes. The man should sleep with her five days after she has finished menstruating."

The stipulation in the last sentence regarding intercourse on the tenth day from the start of a menstrual period might actually render this medicine effective since the change of conception would then be at its highest.

The contents of the second book, from the hands of an Ibadan man, has a preface which is more in the nature of frank advertisement. "We beg you," says the author, "if you buy this book to preserve it carefully because it is one of the medicine books that belonged to our ancestors. They used it and it has always proved successful. Fortune has come to you! Take and taste it, it is honey and salt." This book contains the details of 50 different medicines. Twenty-one of these (42%) relate to sexual and reproductive functions or to child care.

Pre-occupations with potency and success in love are understandable among the mainly male readership of a manual of this sort. The ten remedies or potions in this category are as follows:

"1. Remedy to cure Máágun. (A generally fatal condition widely believed to follow inevitably upon adultery. The illness, if it does occur, may be an example of what has been called "magic fright", induced by auto-suggestion.)
2. Medicine to compel a woman to run into your house.
3. Incantation for inducing a girl to have sexual dealings with you.
4. Medicine for an unfaithful woman.
5. Medicine to win the love of a girl.
6. Incantation for gonorrhoea.
7. Incantation to help deflower a virgin.
8. Incantation to be used when a man encounters a woman for intercourse just after she has finished menstruating.
9. Medicine to stiffen the penis.
10. Medicine to help a man produce more semen."

There are seven references to pregnancy and fertility:
"1. Remedy to help a woman deliver in a case of complicated pregnancy.
2. Medicine to help a woman become pregnant.
3. Medicine to make a woman productive.
4. Medicine to clean the womb of a barren woman.
5. Medicine to make your house full (of children).
6. Incantation to stop (women's) bleeding.
7. Medicine for stomach ache after childbirth."

The following four prescriptions relate to aspects of child care:
"1. Medicine for a child who will not talk.
2. Medicine for a child who is very fat and sickly.
3. Medicine for children who are being molested by their spirit companions (*abiku*).
4. Soap for washing a baby who has just begun to grow teeth."

The interview material in the study showed how Yoruba women were still prepared to try alternative methods for ensuring fertility and for helping them through the trials of pregnancy and labour. Someone fearing the curse and consequences of childlessness is likely to seek all kinds of advice from invocation of the gods, through consultations with various traditional diviners and herbalists and even with Western trained obstetricians and psychiatrists. There was no significant difference between town and country dwellers in their tendency to consult with traditional practitioners on the questions of fertility and infertility. Infertility is a matter of central importance to society as well as to the individual or family.

Once conception has been achieved, the townswoman in Ibadan today has the chance to obtain modern antenatal care, although she may still decide to choose the older methods. Women may use medicines from both sources, as a double insurance against misfortune. Modern facilities for hospital delivery are well patronized in places where distance does not preclude easy attendance at clinics and where the reputation for good care has been established.

The persistent patronage of traditional specialists for matters to do with fertility is explicable in terms of its significance for the continuance of the group. But an event like a pregnancy following upon a consultation with a local healer will easily be attributed to the remedy and to the observance prescribed by someone who is already inclined to belief. Even in the setting of Western medicine, problems of infertility, relative or absolute, are notoriously difficult to resolve and it is often impossible to attribute with certainty a subsequent pregnancy to one particular regimen or drug.

Once a Yoruba child is born it faces a multiplicity of hazards, some of which are compounded by the procedures accompanying home delivery, especially the use of dirty dressings for the umbilicus. Mothers of most cultures are alert to the greatly heightened dangers of the immediate postnatal period and take refuge in all kinds of magical rituals as well as in medical precautions. In the Nigerian situation, modern medical care for infants and small children is steadily enhancing its reputation, particularly among the younger women. The women who use or have used traditional medicines for their children tend to be older and nowadays younger women are prepared to defy their elders over this issue and go to hospitals for paediatric advice. It seems as though the manifest advantages of antibiotics, dietary supplements, intravenous fluids and so on, are rapidly appreciated by mothers whose prime concern is to receive rapid and effective treatment for their desperately ill children.

Conception may or may not be due to a particular medicine or special method, there is room for doubt about this, but a sick infant who does not receive prompt effective treatment will surely die. Yoruba mothers are empiricists, prepared to accept methods which are patently successful. The successes and continued popularity of African medicine lie primarily in the realm of adult illness, where chronicity and an element of psychosomatic effect can both sustain belief in the efficacy of specific treatments, magical or herbal. Many folk remedies for children are definitely harmful, if not actually contaminated they may contain powerful irritants which can induce fatal dehydration. The dosage of potent plant constituents is largely uncontrolled.

Yoruba mothers persist in their rationalization of multiple child deaths by the touching belief in *abiku* children. This fatalism offers some kind of defence in the face of a high infantile mortality; yet it is not completely fatalistic, as is shown by the names which mothers give to children whom they believe to be *abiku*.

There is also a lingering belief in the possibility of stimulating lactation in a woman who is called upon to suckle an orphaned child. There has not been any serious research to discover whether there is a basis for this belief.

The Ibadan healers who were studied were mainly middle aged or elderly men, which might suggest that they are dying out. But, on the other hand, they reported long apprenticeships and they are now trying to make a stand in the face of modern competition by advertisements, by joining together in associations and, in some cases, by privately publishing their most popular remedies. They all reported a great many consultations regarding matters to do with reproduction and child care. The two booklets briefly referred to gave ample evidence of the prominence of recipes for success in love, for ensuring conception and for dealing with women's ailments.

However, this whole area requires much more research. A first essential is the establishment of a simple register of births and deaths. This could be the responsibility of a medical assistant or dispensary attendant in rural areas. This would give a picture of changing infant and maternal mortality, provided it could be tied to local census figures. It is also desirable to have more information on the experience and behaviour of women over an entire period of childbearing, which children they choose to deliver in hospital and why. What was the outcome of successive pregnancies and what reasons did women give for what happened to them? How widespread is the practice of female circumcision and how does it affect their sexual capacity and enjoyment or their menstrual functioning? What advantages and disadvantages are seen by women themselves to pertain to (a) traditional, home confinements, (b) hospital confinements or (c) confinement in a small rural centre? There is also much scope for the introduction of improved basic skills to local women who may be called upon to assist their sisters in labour. It would be wrong to criticize those who are largely without choice in the matter of childbearing and childrearing. They could at least be helped towards achieving healthy infants who have better chances of survival than previous generations.

Notes

(1) One of the plants in common use is known by the Yoruba name *amunimuye*. It contains senecio alkaloids which are liver poisons.
(2) There are also a number of alternative umbilical dressings, all carrying a very high risk of neo-natal tetanus, a common cause of early death. Puerperal sepsis from these dressings is not unusual, too.
(3) In fact, the protein deficiency disease, *kwashiorkor*, does affect the child weaned to make way for another.
(4) A poorly nourished Yoruba mother often fails to breast-feed both infants successfully. Marasmic babies would be brought to hospital, contrasting starkly with a plump sibling.

References

Ajose, O. A. (1957). "Preventive Medicine and Superstition in Nigeria". *Africa* **27**, 268–274.

Atalabi, G. (1964). "Cow's Urine Poisoning: An Account of a Widely Used Traditional Remedy in Yorubaland". *Dokita* (Journal of Ibaden University Medical Students) **61**, 1–4.

Barber, C. R. (1966). "An Enquiry into Possible Social Factors Making for Acceptance of Institutional Delivery in a Predominantly Rural Area of Western Nigeria". *Journal of Tropical Medicine and Hygiene* **69**, 63–65.

Idowu, E. B. (1962). *Oledumare: God in Yoruba Belief*. London: Longmans.

Jahn, J. (1962). "Afrikanische Medizin". *Therapie des Monats* **12**, 54–64 and 100–112.

Jelliffe, D. B. and Jelliffe, E. F. P. (1977). "The Infant Food Industry and International Child Health". *International Journal of Health Services* **7**, 249–254.

Lambo, T. A. (1956). "Neuropsychiatric Observations in the Western Region of Nigeria". *British Medical Journal* **ii**, 1388–1394.

Lambo, T. A. (1964). "The Village of Aro". *Lancet* **i**, 513–514.

Lawson, J. B. and Stewart, D. B. (1967). *Obstetrics and Gynaecology in the Tropics and Developing Countries*. London: Edward Arnold.

Little, K. (1966). *West African Urbanization: A Study of Voluntary Associations in Social Change.* Cambridge: Cambridge University Press.

Lloyd, P. C. (1967). *Africa in Social Change.* Harmondsworth: Penguin.

Maclean, C. M. U. (1965). "Tradition in Transition". *British Journal of Preventive and Social Medicine* **19**, 192–197.

Maclean, C. M. U. (1966). "Hospitals or Healers? An Attitude Survey in Ibadan". *Human Organization* **25**, 131–139.

Maclean, C. M. U. (1969a). "In Defence of their Children". *New Society*, 10 July 1969, 52–54.

Maclean, C. M. U. (1969b). "Traditional Healers and Their Female Clients: An Aspect of Nigerian Sickness Behaviour". *Journal of Health and Social Behaviour* **10**, 172–186.

Maclean, C. M. U. (1971). *Magical Medicine: A Nigerian Case Study.* London: Allan Lance.

Parrinder, G. (1953). *Religion in an African City.* Oxford: Oxford University Press.

Verger, P. (1957). "Notes sur la culte des Orisa et Vodun". *Memoires de l'Institut Francais d'Afrique Noire*, No. 51.

Verger, P. (1966). "Tranquillizers and Stimulants in Yoruba Pharmaceuticals". Mimeographed copy of paper read to Ibadan University Seminar on Traditional Medical Practice.

World Health Organization (1978). *The Promotion and Development of Traditional Medicine.* Technical Report Series No. 662. Geneva: WHO.

7. The Social Context of Birth: Some Comparisons between Childbirth in Jamaica and Britain

S. KITZINGER

Comparative study of childbirth in Jamaica and Britain suggests that all analyses of physiological states should focus on the dynamic interaction between meaning systems, social behaviour and physiological functions. Birth, like death, is not only a physiological fact but also a social act. Entrance into and exit from the social system is the signal for a realignment of existing relationships and the building of new ones, and provides a focus for highly significant social values.

Within a Western frame of reference, we tend to view birth from the standpoint of our own technological orientation which is concerned with gaining control over natural processes, eliminating pain and reducing mortality. This view is historically rooted in the Victorian "calling" to improve all institutions of "primitive" society. But a true comparative sociology must see our own culture of childbirth in both historical and cross-cultural comparative terms and not simply take it as a given vantage point. For the study of birth to be comparative there must be comparable data and a generally accepted terminology to describe what is observed. Nor is it enough simply to record posture, medications, midwifery manoeuvres and data of this kind. A multidimensional approach is required in which birth is seen as operating with a specific social context and a particular value system, involving interaction between individuals and groups in defined relationships.

Birth as a Rite of Passage

If we view birth as a rite of passage, the patterns of interaction between individuals and social groups comes clearly into focus. Transitional rites· define and regulate the passage from one social status to another. They guard the threshold between social categories of being. The individual on the journey between two kinds of social identity is controlled and protected and the behaviour of everyone involved carefully circumscribed to achieve an orderly transition.

Transition rites consist of separation, trial and re-entry in a newly defined social state. With separation, the initiate is physically and symbolically set apart from peers and removed to a different place. He or she is often divested of accustomed personal attributes, including any belongings which differentiate the individual, such as clothing and name. Washing, purging and other symbolic representations of being set apart from everyday life, cleansed and renewed, are further elements in the drama. In many of these rites the initiate goes through an act of infantilization, in which he or she is reduced to the state of a small, dependent, submissive child. The initiate's body is often manipulated and he or she must passively accept what is done. It is as if only by going back to the beginning can re-birth take place.

Pregnancy taboos, dietary rules for the expectant mother, "old wives' tales" in our own society, the highly formalized and circumscribed interaction of the hospital booking clinic by which pregnancy is given public recognition, can all be seen as parts of rites of status transformation. Baptism, circumcision, naming ceremonies, segregation of the new mother and baby, churching of women, taboos on sexual intercourse following birth, even the postnatal check-up are all often complicated steps in a kind of dance which continues until mother and child are safely established in their correct social places and are considered no longer at risk. The concept of "at risk" is basic to such rites, for the transition between different social identities is believed to be fraught with peril, not only for the individual on the journey but also for the social group in which the upheaval is taking place. An essential element in the drama is that all those participating believe in the danger.

Such rituals may support the individual and the kin group across the bridge into a new social state, but it is probably wrong to see their main function as that of providing emotional support. In fact, they reinforce an established social system. Hospital systems have rituals for recognizing a status of illness. They turn people into patients who no longer do ordinary activities, divest them of their usual rights and responsibilities and take them through a process of healing to the status of health. In large centralized, hierarchical institutions existing outside and apart from the family there is special likelihood of these rituals being used to reinforce the existing system and maintain the power structure. In pregnancy each culture has its own transitional ceremonies and draws its own map, as it were, of significant points and milestones to which behaviour is linked.

In those hospitals where "active management of labour" is the preferred policy, the woman has a catheter inserted in a vein of the arm through which a synthetic hormone is steadily dripped to augment labour. She is connected to a continuous foetal monitor, the electrodes of which are strapped to her abdomen or inserted through the vagina and clipped or screwed onto the baby's scalp which record the pressure of each contraction and every foetal heartbeat.

There is usually limited possibility of movement since the catheter is easily dislodged and the electrodes disturbed. To discover how long and powerful the contractions are, doctors and midwives look at the print-out from the monitor rather than asking the mother (Kitzinger, 1978, pp. 142–162). Epidural anaesthesia may be given before or after acceleration of labour. This removes most sensation from the waist down and allows oxytocin to be used regardless of the pain it would otherwise cause. The woman cannot move her legs and must be turned by attendants and have her bladder emptied by a catheter. Once epidural anaesthesia is given staff can concentrate on recording data rather than giving care. Many women, even those who are concerned to be "good patients", indicate that they feel alienated from their bodies and deprived of autonomy under such conditions.

Now that the patient has been processed the husband is allowed in, heavily garbed against danger of contagion to mother and baby (Roth, 1957). He is often given instructions in interpreting the monitor readings and readily becomes interested in the machinery. Interaction between husband and wife is always regulated by the social context in which the birth takes place. In high technology hospital labours it tends to be reduced to the minimum except in those cases where one or more staff members thinks it important.

One question that might be asked about modern hospital rituals is whether the rites have become so professionalized and stressful for women undergoing them that re-entry into society as a mother is thereby made unnecessarily difficult. The incidence of postnatal depression, which has been estimated as affecting up to 25% of all mothers, and of postpartum anxiety and child abuse throughout Western society (Kaij and Nilsson, 1972; Kempe, 1978) suggests that a highly complex variety of rites serves largely to reinforce the medical care system, maintaining the structure of the hospital institution and the relative status of those in it (Goffman, 1971, 1972), rather than supporting the women who are becoming mothers and the families into which the babies are being born (see Jones, Chapter 10).

Babies are often separated from their mothers for some or all of the hospital stay in communal nurseries. Women who have their babies beside their beds may be instructed not to cuddle their babies or to take them into bed with them (Kitzinger, 1979). Babies who require skilled care may be put, as a matter of routine, into special care units, a procedure which in effect tells a mother that she is not good enough to care for the baby (Richards, 1978).

Feeding times may be regulated by the clock, fathers and older siblings treated as dangerous carriers of bacteria and potential threats to baby's welfare, and new mothers expected to be dependent on professional advice and to relate to their babies only under expert direction at certain designated times and in the mode accepted as normal on that particular postpartum ward.

Jamaican Case Study

In a society which grew out of the institution of slavery, fertility was vital in order to replenish the labour force. For the Jamaican girl, as in many other peasant societies, childbirth provides ritual entry to adult state. Adulthood does not come so much with age or experience as with motherhood. When a girl has borne a child she is considered to be a "big woman". The woman who has not had a child is despised as a "mule", a term which dates from slavery, when the infertile female slave was an uneconomic proposition for the plantation owner. It is in this context that pseudocyesis is reported by midwives to occur frequently, particularly in rural areas, and that some 16- and 17-year-olds who have not conceived go to clinics afraid that they are barren. If one cannot have children oneself, one fosters other people's children.

Norms of female beauty are linked to fertility. One element in the peasant ideal is a generously sized pelvis and well-padded buttocks. It is a compliment to tell a woman that she has big hips. Young women out to catch a man adopt the "Africa walk", best performed in a skintight skirt, slit up one side, emphasizing the hips and under-carriage. The walk consists of an exaggerated pelvic movement with the upper thighs held close together with a rolling gait.

In spite of the value of fertility in the peasant society there is growing political and social pressure in modern Jamaica to "space between" (the peasant term for contraception) or to "stop altogether" (sterilization). This involves a radical change in values concerning the family and female roles.

In group discussions with adolescent girls still at school I asked: "Do you want your lives to be the same as your mother's or different in any way?" Though some said they wanted to be different, the only way they could envisage an alternative life style was to have a job before they had babies. Those few who did not want to bear children themselves said they would "adopt". A life without a man is just conceivable, but it is difficult for a Jamaican woman to imagine one without children. A woman has little hope of getting a man to marry her or to accept economic responsibility unless she has a child. She is said to bear a child "for" a man. The real testing time for a conjugal relationship comes after the birth, when the man makes implicit recognition of paternity by remaining with the mother. If he accepts social fatherhood, whether or not he is the biological father, the union is put onto a more solid basis and the woman acquires additional status as having a consort.

Should a woman be still in her mother's or grandmother's home or living alone, if she can get the father to "response" for the child, even only to the extent of a single cash payment, the baby is given that man's surname. If she cannot get him to accept responsibility, the child is registered with her surname. Thus a woman often has several children with different surnames, including her own. Occasionally, if everyone in the neighbourhood knows, or thinks they know the father, the child is given his name even if he refuses to "response" for it. This naming of the child acts as a social sanction to encourage payment.

Man and Woman, Mother and Daughter

Pregnancy in the adolescent girl is not greeted with joy, but derision and anger, on the part of her parents. The exceptions are when the girl, though unmarried, has a man who will "response" for the baby and accept social paternity. The ideal but rarely realized behaviour code is that the young man should formally visit the girl's mother and ask her permission to be "in friendship" with her, indicating at the same time that he has the wherewithal to provide economic support and "stand manly". Parents do not always agree to a union. One woman who had five children before she married said that the father of the first child went to tell her parents that he had "bred" her, but her mother said the fellow was black and I should "take somebody fairer than me. The old time people were more up on quality".

The young man is anxious to become a father, for it is parenthood and having a child "named for" him that ultimately proves his virility, not simply the fact that he "grinds" girls. Men are proud of the children they have, and tend to add on the ones that die or even those who were miscarried, just as women do. But often they are unwilling or unable because of unemployment and poverty to take on economic responsibility.

My main study, in association with the Medical Research Council Epidemiology Unit, was carried out in a rural area. In many family units, the men resided uxorilocally on a small plot of land owned by the wife's family. Many men were unemployed and the family subsisted on produce from the small holding. Women sold plaited straw mats and "higgled" (traded) surplus produce. Men are often caught up in a very complicated pattern of economic responsibility to children they have fathered on different women, those with whom they are or have been living and others who are born of visiting unions. Approximately one-third of women have consorts living with them who pay towards the support of "outside" children. Stycos and Back (1947, pp. 332–339) remark that

> a remarkably consistent picture of adjustments of the family system to the exigencies of the fluid pattern of mating and childbearing emerges, a system in which resources are pooled in order to provide economic and child-rearing support for children occurring out of wedlock.

When a woman suspects that her daughter is "with stomach", behaviour is heavily ritualized. She first asks her, "Who trouble you then?" and questions her to find whose stomach it is. If the boy is named she may go to see him and there is a public dispute involving neighbours in which the boy's mother is one of the chief protagonists. She says that "the girl has been bother her son"; the ritualized exchange is crystallized in a calypso:

> Keep your daughter inside Miss Miriam
> That girl child looking for trouble.
> If my boy child trouble your girl child,
> Doan' hold me responsible.

There is a "quarrel" between mother and daughter in the public arena of the mud yard outside the house. The mother or mother's consort flogs her with a strap and turns her out of the house. This ritual quarrel marks social disapproval not of extra-marital sex, nor of illegitimacy, but of reproduction without paternal obligations. At this point, female maternal kin are also involved and the girl often goes to her "aunty's" (mother's sister or other maternal relative) for anything from a few days to several months. Towards the end of her pregnancy or after the birth the girl is usually received back into her maternal home with her baby. She is now "grown up". It is as if she has passed a test and has crossed over the bridge into adulthood by virtue of her suffering and by accepting responsibility as a mother (Kitzinger, 1978, p. 221).

Although there may be friction initially, in peasant Jamaica birth also has a cohesive function. When the adolescent girl becomes pregnant, women of the neighbourhood come together to share the information, discuss the right course to follow and pass judgement on the girl and her mother. Rural Jamaican dwellings in the hills are highly dispersed; villages are few and far between and the land is dotted with small holdings which are mere clearings in the bush each with its own wood and corrugated-iron shack. Neighbours meet at church, at the weekly market in the town, and when washing clothes at the nearest available supply of water, standpipe, river or gulley. The rumour of a first pregnancy (the postmistress and the midwife are primary sources of information) is an occasion for exchange of information and draws women together. One or more of these women later acts as mediator between mother and daughter and persuades the mother to take her daughter back again.

Mothers often rear their daughter's firstborn, and sometimes subsequent children too, and the unity of the maternal family across the generations is thus asserted through obligations of reciprocity between mothers and daughters. The girl has achieved maturity and because there is then one more mouth to feed, putting the family under further economic pressure, goes off to work. Since opportunities for wage employment are severely limited in rural areas, she usually goes to the town or may emigrate. She hands the child over to her mother with an understanding that she will provide financial help. It is a pattern of exchange which forms the basis of a social system in which the object exchanged is the fruit of the uterus.

This ritual transaction seals the bond between mother and daughter in a new and indissoluble way. Even when adult the woman remains dependent on her mother for emotional support, financial assistance and practical help. Every other relationship is less reliable. In some way this mother–daughter bond is the model for all relations between women, for there exists a wider network of reciprocal obligations between women which creates the primary social cohesion of Jamaican peasant society.

Nana: the Midwife

The nana or folk midwife is a key figure in the cohesion of women in Jamaican rural communities. Nanas are women of high standing and great authority, though their time-sanctioned and customary calling is not legally recognized in modern Jamaica. The triad of the postmistress, the school teacher and the nana traditionally forms the political centre of each community, controls the channels of communication within it, and between it and the larger society, and presides over the main transitional rites in each individual life cycle

Channels for social mobility are very restricted in peasant communities. Most positions of high status entail educational qualifications, but the nana role bypasses formal qualifications. It overlaps with the ritual role of women in cult groups. Nanas tend also to be active members of revivalist churches and charismatic leaders in the experience of spirit possession. Eight of the 11 nanas whom I interviewed were central figures in their church and this gave an extra dimension of authority to their midwifery role.

The word "nana" was that used for the "grandmothers" who cared for the children of slaves while their mothers worked in the plantation. Nanas were primarily grandmother figures. Being elderly, they are a link with the ancestors, shepherding people between the spirit and the human worlds and guarding the threshold. The aptitude and skills of the nana tend to be handed down from mother to daughter. Nowadays, this may mean that the daughter goes off to train as a nurse and midwife. Nine of the 11 nanas I interviewed had daughters who were training in British or other hospitals abroad. Within rural communities, however, skills are assessed by results and it is only possible for a woman to be accepted as a nana if the outcome for mothers and babies in her care is seen to be good.

No one can become a nana until she has borne children herself. To be a nana is really an extension of the mothering role, so all nanas are mothers who are seen to be successful in their role. Their social esteem is expressed in the term by which they are addressed which is "mistress", a title otherwise restricted to married women. They are also neighbourly women, willing to lend a hand and help out in times of family crisis and, above all, are social facilitators. The first request to help at a birth is in the nature of a trial and if all goes well and her client likes her others will also engage her services.

For many members of the Jamaican middle class, nanas are evil old busy-bodies who kill almost as many as they help and who are opposed to every benefit conferred on Jamaica by science and medicine, embarrassing symbols of customs associated with slavery and subjection. Yet I met many labouring women in a Kingston hospital who bemoaned the fact that they were not in the country under a nana's care because they believed the nana knew how to make women more comfortable in labour, had superior means of pain relief, encouraged them more and was able to make the birth easier. Women often compared the labour in hospital with that with the nana and felt neglected and denied understanding support from the hospital midwives.

There is inherent conflict between the medical profession, pioneers of asepsis and order, on the one hand, and the folk midwives who do things "the old time way". If a woman haemorrhages the nana either calls in the trained midwife (and if she does not wish to leave her client then poses as a relative), or sends the woman to hospital. Professionals, therefore, believe that the practices of nanas result in haemorrhage, though since they only see cases in which there is haemorrhage this inference is probably false. The incidence of tetanus neonatorum in babies delivered by nanas is also said to be high. Any attempt to incorporate nanas into organized health care has been met with suspicion by professionals, though nanas themselves have sometimes felt threatened by an alien technology. An epidemiologist taught nanas how to weigh and measure babies for his study and at the same time showed them how to sterilize scissors with which they cut the cord. The nanas co-operated gladly, but he was accused by colleagues of trying to train an inferior category of health worker and the project was dropped.

If nanas have an opportunity, they are eager to watch how trained midwives conduct deliveries. They are also eager to read, or have read to them, midwifery textbooks from Britain. They are highly motivated to learn as much as they can and are grateful for any recognition and approval they are offered.

It is now being acknowledged that traditional midwives have a positive role to play but need help if they are to be integrated into an evolving health service (WHO, 1979). Because of their empirical knowledge, their understanding of indigenous values and their position at a focal point of rural communications, they have an especially important function in preventive health during pregnancy. It should be the responsibility of health services to prepare them, wherever possible, to take an active part in community-centred health care.

As many as 25% of Jamaican babies may be delivered by nanas, especially in rural areas, though such births are registered as "born unattended" or "delivered by mother" (or by a friend or relative). Even if the woman books the trained midwife for delivery she may ask the nana to attend her during the first stage of labour and throughout pregnancy. The care given by the nana continues through pregnancy, labour and for nine days after the birth. Her role is to conduct the woman and baby safely through pregnancy, birth and the postpartum period. The bringing to life of the baby is seen as a process through which a woman needs to be shepherded, and though the birth is a dramatic event it is not usually conceived of as a medical crisis. When talking about the total experience women often complain far more of the discomforts and trials of pregnancy than of any pain and distress in labour.

Pregnancy

Because the pregnant woman is in a state of transition, bringing to birth another individual who is undergoing the same dangerous transitional process, she is in ritual danger from which she is protected only through the careful observances of taboos. The nana guards her and helps her through this passage.

The most important taboos involve the strict separation of the principles of life and death. No pregnant woman must look at a dead body. Though she can be present when a body is lying in the "booth" at a "set-up" for the dead she must on no account look at it. The younger the mother the more vulnerable she is. If she does see a corpse her blood is chilled to the temperature of the corpse's: "Your body get cold. Energy leave you", and this results in the death of the baby and also sometimes of the mother, either immediately or when she is in labour. Nor must a pregnant woman hold another woman's baby under the age of three months or the child inside her will die.

The nana teaches strict dietary regulations. If the pregnant woman drinks too much water she will "drown" the baby. (There seems to be recognition here of the association between hydramnios and poor foetal outcome.) The pregnant woman should avoid stretching her arms above her head lest "the baby's neck scorch". She must not walk over a floor which is being scrubbed with soap or she will get indigestion, nor step over a donkey's tethering rope or a broom lest the pregnancy be prolonged. She should not become emotionally disturbed or the child can be "marked": "If you killing a fowl and you sorrow for that fowl your child come with some parts of the looks belonging to the fowl". For this reason a pregnant woman should never wring a chicken's neck. Nanas sometimes smile over these prohibitions and pride themselves on being up-to-date. Nevertheless, they give tacit support to the myths existing in the culture and explain that, for example, the prohibition on using a treadle sewing machine in advanced pregnancy is useful because many women sit long hours over their machines and get severe backache as a result.

Pregnant women are vulnerable to the activities of the duppies (ancestor spirits). They can lay hands on the baby *in utero* and make it sicken and die. Eclampsia is seen as spirit possession, the duppies having taken over the soul of the sick woman. So many pre-eclamptic patients had seen duppies haunting their ward in the public maternity hospital in Kingston that it had to be moved to another floor of the building. The nana tells pregnant women to eat plenty of callalu (a vegetable like spinach) to enrich the blood. Okra makes the baby slide out, since its slippery inner surfaces are thought to grease the passage. Women are also told to eat oranges and to drink bush teas. The recommended teas are "bitters", in particular cerasee, which "cools" the blood.

Sexual intercourse during pregnancy "nourishes" the womb and also keeps the birth canal open so that delivery is easy. A nana explained to a woman that her labour was difficult because she had not had intercourse during pregnancy and so was "closed".

In everything the pregnant woman must be careful, deliberate, free from anxiety and from emotional extremes, active but not overworked, eating moderately and behaving with circumspection. When the nana takes a woman under care she accepts responsibility for guiding her in this way over the bridge into motherhood.

For a small payment in cash or kind the nana visits the expectant mother at intervals through pregnancy to counsel her and, using oil from the wild castor oil plant or olive oil, to massage her abdomen and "shape the baby". She usually knows her and her family well even before the pregnancy starts but frequent visits mean that the two are in an intimate relationship by the time the labour begins. Most nanas do not charge the very poor. After the delivery they care for mother and baby and for any other children of the family, and do the house-keeping, washing and shopping until the mother is ready to take over. In this they are assisted by the mother's female kin, and the women work together in a shared enterprise in much the same way as did the "gossips" of mediaeval England when attending a lying-in.

Labour and Birth

A basic Jamaican concept of ill-health is that a passage or orifice is blocked and the cure consists of releasing the blockage. The nana sees her primary function as that of "freeing" the mother's body for birth. Everything she does is designed to facilitate the natural process, to "bring on the pains in front", to "let it open gradual", to "give them good words and cheer them up so that they will soon get deliverance".

Nanas advise their clients to walk around during labour and the two women together light the stove, fetch water and set it to boil, make the bed up with newspapers, tear up rags in which to wrap the baby and make the cornmeal porridge which is the customary food for after delivery. During contractions in the late first stage the nana massages the mother's lower abdomen and sometimes in the second stage massages the perineum, with olive or castor oil or the oil from toona leaves. Hot compresses are also used. Herbal teas are given, especially thyme and spice teas for uterine inertia and prolonged labour. If delivery is delayed and a sweat-soaked shirt of the baby's father can be obtained, the mother is urged to take deep breaths of this to accelerate labour. There is a high concentration of prostaglandins in human sweat.

Nanas perform external versions of breech births and sometimes, when there is a posterior presentation, use massage to rotate the head to the anterior. Some send the mother to hospital if they are unable to turn a breech; others deliver a breech, allowing the baby's body to hang by its own weight, and raise the legs up over the mother's pubis to deliver the aftercoming head.

For treating backache the nana uses a band of cotton cloth of approximately a fore-arm's width, which she extends round the mother's sacrolumbar region and, facing her patient, pulls this cloth alternately from side to side during contractions to produce strong friction. If labour is hard some nanas wrap the mother in hot, wet towels and when the skin is warm, remove them and massage the entire body with olive oil.

Nanas tell women to breathe lightly in the late first stage. It is believed that the baby can ascend into the mother's chest and "by inhaling more the baby come up". The nanas are well aware that this cannot happen but use the myth to encourage their clients to breathe shallowly and quickly: "Too much hearty breathing gives bad sensations", a reference to hyper-ventilation.

In the second stage of labour a helper or the woman's consort is often called in to support the mother's back so that she sits up for delivery, legs apart and feet on the bed. If other children are in the bed a washing line may be suspended down the length of the bed and a cloth thrown over it, separating them from the labouring woman, and the nana holds the baby up over the screen to show the children immediately. Prolonged breath-holding and straining is discouraged. As Mistress Wilhel, an experienced nana who kept an "accounter book" with details of more than 2000 labours she had attended since 1927, explained, "You push gentle and you give a little rest and you push again. Pushing hard brings on weakness".

At delivery the nana lays the baby on its front on the mother's abdomen and does not cut the cord until it stops pulsating, and often in fact, leaves it until after the placenta is delivered. If the baby is not breathing well she holds the baby's head down and "milks" mucus from the nose by pinching the nostrils and then blows cigarette smoke on to its anterior fontanelle, "mole". If there is bleeding in the third stage the nana instructs the mother to take a deep breath and then blow into a bottle, which causes pressure on the fundus and tends to produce strong uterine contractions. The mother's vulva is cleaned by her squatting over a bucket of steaming water "hot like nine days love". The baby is washed in cold water tinted with washing blue to keep away the duppies. The cord stump is treated with grated nutmeg mixed with powder, and a binder is put on. Nutmeg has antiseptic qualities and is slightly irritant so causing the cord to slough off early. The nana massages the baby with coconut or olive oil. It is often given a pre-lacteal feed of jack-in-the-bush or mint tea, three drops of castor oil are put on its tongue to make it cough up any further mucus and it is then put to the breast.

Postpartum Period

A period of ritual seclusion follows birth. Traditionally this period of intense seclusion is supposed to last for nine nights, the same as after a death. A secondary, less restricted period of seclusion lasts 40 nights from delivery.

During the first period the woman remains with her baby in the darkness of the hut, windows or shutters tightly closed, under the care of the "grandy" (her mother) and the nana. She wears a turban over her hair lest she get "baby cold", which is said to cause deafness and paralysis. She must refrain from all household chores while the bones of her lower spine, which it is believed must swing open like a gate for the baby to be born, "knit up".

The baby lies on her bed wearing some red garment. By the bed is a Bible open at the twenty-third psalm, a pair of scissors and a tape measure. These precautions keep the duppies away. The most important rule of conduct is that the baby must not be allowed to cry, but must be put to the breast as it stirs from sleep, for duppies are attracted to come to play with the baby and may be unable to let the child go, causing it to sicken and die. A baby who is weak or pre-term has a talisman tied round its neck or pinned to its clothing containing a silver coin, garlic, grain and oesyphetida which may also be rubbed into the baby's hair. Should the baby die, the same "nine nights" are observed, and the seclusion is terminated by the mother taking a broom and sweeping the reality of the baby out of the hut. If she fails to do this the spirit of the child may come back as a duppy to haunt the home.

At the end of the "ny night" mother and baby emerge, but only when the sun is high. The baby is often put in a scrubbed washing bucket under the shade of a tree on the mud patch outside the dwelling while the mother does her household tasks. She still observes dietary taboos: rice is not eaten lest she conceive again too soon. Some food, fruit and chewed sugarcane, must be eaten only at mid-day or they can affect her milk and give the baby gripe. At the end of the liminal period of 40 days the mother unwraps her turban and washes her hair, so making the entry into a new phase of existence.

In fact, the exigencies of life and poverty cut short these liminal periods of seclusion and carefulness for most peasant women. But, not withstanding, correct behaviour at birth and post partum is considered important and is integrated into a system of values which is shared by all the participants. The nana has a central and vitally important role in shepherding those involved through the drama of what is essentially the re-birth of a woman as a mother.

The Symbolic Value of Birth

Levi-Strauss reminds us that birth and death are rich with meanings which have penetrated the whole of social life. But in the West, as part of a process of "scientific praxis", he feels we have emptied birth and death of everything not corresponding to mere physiological processes, rendering them unsuitable to convey other meanings (1966, p. 264). Meanings of birth and death are expressed in the symbolic medium of language, but in the West a gulf exists between the language birth professionals use and that used by ordinary people. Is a pregnant woman really a "patient" or a "woman"? Obstetricians speak of birth as "delivery", connoting an act done to a patient by the professional birth operator. A different meaning is conveyed in the term "birthing", a process in which the mother herself is active.

The meaning of birth is embedded within larger value systems. This is expressed in verbal and visual symbolism, one form of which is the metaphor of the culturally anticipated dream. The Jamaican woman expects a special kind of dream when pregnant. This dream legitimizes the pregnancy and, as it were, makes of it a psychic as well as an everyday reality. Some women will not acknowledge a pregnancy until they have had this fertility dream. Others accept that they are pregnant but do not feel comfortable about it till they have had the dream. I learned about it when I asked, "Do you have dreams when you are pregnant?", a question which in a group of English expectant mothers usually elicit accounts of disturbing dreams some of which have the force and persistence of recurrent nightmares. Among Jamaican peasant women, however, this particular dream marking the acceptance of pregnancy is usually experienced as positive and provides confirmation of the suspected state of pregnancy.

Such dreams include images of ripe fruit bursting with seed, such as melons or paw-paw, or teeming fish. They may also involve a visitation by a dead female relative, particularly from the woman's mother: "I dream me dead mother. I dream that she was pregnant and I dream her in a full white dress". A typical dream of this kind is, "I was lost and two women take me home, but I had to pass through a pasture with a lot of cows. I was afraid. But one of them told me that the cows can't hurt me while she was there. She took me home quite safe. I feel that it was my mother—she's dead four years—and my grandmother". Such dreams may also represent the traditional nature of pregnancy in symbolic form: "I dream about travelling and crossing bridges. When I get on a bridge the bridge go down, but I . . . escape and find myself on the other side". Obeah men and women (sorcerers) are able to interpret these dreams and if a woman is uncertain as to the meaning of her dream or wants to know whether it contains a prophesy she may go to the "balm yard" to consult the Obea man. Her entry into pregnancy is thus not a mere physiological occurrence but a ritual state and one which involves the spirit world.

The congregations of hill revivalist sects in Jamaica are mostly women, called "sisters" or "shepherdesses", and the active worship which consists of dancing and singing in order to enter the state of spirit possession and to speak with tongues is done almost exclusively by them. A lighted candle and a beaker of water are placed on the ground in the centre of the moving circle of women. Candle and water are symbols of the spirit which, since the experience sought is one of rebirth, we may interpret also as representing phallus and amniotic fluid. The women gyrate around these sacred objects with pronounced pelvic movements as they became ecstatic, reiterating "Lahd! Lahd! *Jesus! Jesus!*" with sharp exhalations of breath followed by quick breaths in. As the tempo increases the speed of breathing also increases so that overbreathing and subsequent hyperventilation occur. Resulting peripheral anaesthesia eliminates consciousness of pain when they become possessed by the spirit and fall and roll on the floor. This may be interspersed with short periods of unconsciousness. The process by which this happens is called "labouring".

Tape recordings of these religious services are almost indistinguishable from others I made in the labour wards of a public maternity hospital in Kingston. The same sounds are made, identical words and phrases used and a similar pelvic rocking movement occurs as the woman approaches full dilatation. Women go into hospital with their Bibles so that they can chant passages from the psalms during the first stage. The hospital environment for birth is threatening and they cling to the security they know which is based in revivalist religion. Because the wards are overcrowded so that women must often be two to a bed, they may also cling physically to each other and rock in unison.

In the labour ward religious imagery is used spontaneously by women to describe what they are feeling or to assist their efforts. The analogy between birth and rebirth is implied when a woman shouts "Naked Oh Lord to Thee I Come" or in the second stage pushes exclaiming meanwhile, "Gwan dahn Saviour! Gwan down Lahd", or when she calls on the name of Jesus or chants snatches from the Old Testament in between contractions. The frightening experience of giving birth in the hospital is given meaning and significance by use of powerful symbols drawn from religion, just as the experience of psychic rebirth sought in revivalist services is enhanced by actions associated with the physical sensations of parturition. Symbols of birth and spiritual rebirth are indissolubly linked, metaphorically transformed from one mode into the other and back again (Leach, 1976, pp. 25–27).

Levi-Strauss (1966) has drawn attention in his essay on birth among the Cuna Indians to the way in which the woman's body is thought to be inhabited by spirits which affect physiological function. Muu, the great god of childbirth, dwells in the uterus and may be unwilling to let the child go. The shaman must be called and with his followers makes a mythological journey through the vagina and cervix into the uterus itself, calling on the powers of nature as represented by the woodboring insects and other creatures who can help to free the way for the child to be born. All this is recited in a song saga in the labouring woman's presence. First he describes how careful preparations have been made and assures her that help is at hand. Having entered the uterus and battled with the god, the shaman then reports that whereas they had to come in in single file there is room to walk "three abreast" as they emerge. The cervix is dilating. Here again, we are observing the interdependence of reproductive physiology and the cultural world of meanings. They are not two separate, opposed categories of existence, but one. The same values pervade and the same cosmic forces regulate both.

In Jamaica, in a situation of acute culture conflict, professionals trained in American and British hospitals represent a Western technological style of childbirth while the peasant women giving birth give meaning to the experience by the powerful symbols derived from revivalist religion. The main concern of the nurses and midwives is efficiency, speed of delivery of the patient, hospital routines concerning hygiene and order and the suppression of emotional factors in childbirth so that they can get on with their work in an organized way and treat the greatest number of patients in the shortest possible time. At the time of my research (1965) they encountered almost insuperable obstacles in this: between 35 and 40 women were delivered in each of two eight-bedded delivery rooms every 24 hours. Equipment was always in short supply and was not re-ordered until it had run out. Sterilization of swabs took 48 hours. There was no hot water after early morning, no isolation ward and no means of effectively communicating up the staff hierarchy. In such conditions conflicting expectations of behaviour lead to overt conflict; women would get down off the delivery table and squat, rocking their pelvises and midwives would try to get them back on the table again. One Jamaican labour ward sister asked me "Why do you want to watch them? They are just animals". Doctors and nurses are engaged in a struggle to acquire and maintain control over their patients. Only by the administration of a knockout dose of "the jubilee cocktail" does Western technology at last get its way—and to do so has to mask its barbiturates in Jamaican rum.

In contrast to this, the professionalization of childbirth in Britain is complete and the "active management" of labour is firmly controlled by doctors and midwives, the goal being, in one obstetrician's words, to have every birth taking place "in an intensive care situation" (Whitfield, 1975). Women are for the most part concerned to be "good patients" and doctors' goals become *ipso facto* their goals.

Birth is a medically directed clinical process aimed at the reduction of perinatal mortality rates. Indeed, some obstetricians themselves make an analogy with the organization of professional football, in which it is assumed that spending large amounts of money on expensive facilities and talent inevitably improves position in the league table. In obstetrics "the position in the league" has tended to be purely judged on perinatal mortality figures. Other less easily measured variables, such as effects on relationships in the family and long-term psychosocial outcome, are difficult to quantify and are not usually taken into the reckoning.

Concepts of Sickness and Health

The study of childbirth is one way in which concepts of sickness and health and of the female body can be most clearly understood. Birth puts body percepts in sharp focus because dramatic things happen to the body and its physical boundaries undergo rapid and marked changes in pregnancy, during labour, at delivery and post partum. No other physical transmutation occurs with such speed and on such a large scale except when there is gross mutilation or at death.

Jamaican concepts of sickness are composed of two in some ways disparate body cosmologies, one derived from the mediaeval European "humours" and the other from West African concepts of blockage by objects which, whether by sorcery or other means, have obstructed passages so that body substances can no longer flow. Both these systems meet in the prophylactic treatment of the woman in childbirth and in remedies for ill-health or reproductive malfunctioning. Concepts of humours are implicit in the Jamaican herbal pharmacopeia which is categorized according to the heating or cooling properties of herbs, fruits, vegetables and spices. Spice tea (composed of ginger, cinnamon, nutmeg and other spices as available) is used to "ginger-up" labour and has a mild oxytocic action, according to Waterman (1952). Mint or thyme tea is used to cool the woman in labour when there has been too much "hackling" (hard work/emotional turmoil). A balance must be kept between hot and cold and one of the tasks of the nana is to maintain this precarious balance. As we have seen, she also employs hot and cold substances, "hot stone" on the abdomen or back when there is pain, hot towels wrapped round the woman when she is exhausted, a cold "douse down" should she need cooling.

Another important task is to ensure that the uterus remains in its correct place and does not "come up out of the belly" into the mother's chest, where the baby's hand or fist can choke her. This is related to the body concept in which there is one passage leading between the mouth and the lower orifices, passing through the uterus and the stomach on the way (Kitzinger, 1981). There exists a modern folk mythology about condoms which have come loose and worked their way up to choke women. Nanas themselves do not believe in this mythology, but insist that they must be able to reassure the labouring woman that her uterus is not working up to her chest. In pregnancy the woman wears a tight string under her breasts to keep the baby down, or if she is modern does up her brassiere extra tight instead. In labour the woman who is in a hospital is unlikely to get support or reassurance that the baby is not coming up. The most stressful phase of labour tends to occur at the end of the first stage when the expulsive urge begins to assert itself, initially often experienced as a catch in the throat and an involuntarily held breath. In the context of childbirth in a Jamaican hospital these sensations are taken as an indication that the baby's hand or foot is sticking in her gullet and the woman becomes alarmed.

English middle-class women, in contrast, bring with them into childbirth a body image part of which is a sense of the vagina as tight and unyielding, a constricted passage, pressure on which results in pain and laceration. In talking about their bodies expectant mothers often express the fear that they are "too small down there" or that they will never be able to relax to cope with the sensations of the baby's head as it distends the perineum (Kitzinger, 1976, 1977). They see the vagina not in terms of its concertina-like folds, but as a hard tube controlled by a sphincter like that of the anus. Rectal pressure in the second stage of labour makes the mother feel that she needs to empty her bowels. When this is experienced many women involuntarily contract the musculature of the pelvic floor instead of releasing it so that the baby can be born. Anxiety about defecation and "dirtying the bed" reinforce this active resistance to descent and delivery of the presenting part of the foetus.

The Jamaican peasant mother has the same sensations but is uninhibited by them; she may say "Wanna go do-do" and carries on bearing down without anxiety. In association with such psycho-physiological mechanisms, the second stage is usually short and easy.

Concepts of purity and pollution are interwoven with these culturally variable body ·fantasies which themselves are patterned to represent symbolically values in the social structure. Douglas has pointed out how in the Judaeo-Christian tradition the body is a vessel. Its vital fluids must not be poured away nor diluted and, therefore, its entrances and exits are guarded (Douglas, 1970, p. 130). This is true for many other value systems too. The human body is a symbol of society and represents an organized system of values which must be protected. Pollution is "matter out of place", essentially that which issues from the interior of the body and threatens others with contamination. One aspect of health care and the cure of sickness is how these body products, blood, pus, saliva, faeces, urine, breath and sweat are treated and decharged by society so that they are made safe. In childbirth the blood of the parturient (like menstrual blood), the amniotic fluid, the placenta and the umbilical cord may all have to be decharged in some way if they are not to contaminate men and emasculate them, because of the female essence which they represent.

Physiology, Society and Culture

To understand the meaning of birth and death we must look for dynamic interactions between physiology, society and culture. Physiological and cultural functions are not separate, disparate entities. Eating and drinking and digestion, bowel and bladder movements, opening the body's orifices or keeping them closed, sex and reproductive behaviour, lactation and menstruation are socially controlled physiological activities. In his Cuna Indian essay Levi-Strauss (1967) analyses interaction between meaning systems and social acts, but leaves out physiological functions. He does not tell us how the woman's progress through labour was affected by the song drama.

In our own rapidly changing culture of childbirth the relation between social structure, values and biological variables needs to be explored. In any society a labouring woman's breathing, posture and movements are influenced by the physical environment in which birth takes place, by her relation with her attendants and the instructions they give her, by culturally accepted assumptions about what is happening and the body percepts of all those involved. Emotional reactions (fear, anxiety, joy) may affect physiological function and, specifically, uterine contractility, as a direct consequence of hormone activity—the ratio of adrenaline, for example, which is inhibitory, and noradrenaline, which stimulates nerve endings (Flanders Dunbar, 1946). Emotion also often produces chemical changes in the blood, muscle tension and modification of the heart rate and blood pressure. Because the foetus is completely dependent on the mother, metabolic and other changes in her body affect it. We also need to explore the inter-relation between maternal posture, breathing rates, levels and rhythms customary in labour, the different phases of effacement, dilatation and expulsion, and the biochemical status of mother and foetus.

Integral to this analysis are birth rituals and powerful images such as that of the burst grain jar to release the child from the mother's body or the slowly opening flower which is placed beside the Indian labouring woman to represent the dilatation of the cervix and the progress of labour. We must seek to discover whether there is any association between the kinds of psychological support given in different societies and uterine function.

Integrated physiology and anthropology could examine also the effects of different kinds of culturally approved posture and movement of labour. We know already that the immobile, supine position favoured in Western hospitals in sharp contrast to positions in which the upper part of the labouring woman's body is raised, as in many other societies, tends to result in pressure on the inferior vena cava and reduced blood flow to the foetus (Caldeyro-Barcia *et al.*, 1960), and that a woman lying in bed is likely to have contractions which are less efficient, but more painful, than if she is up and moving around, while at the same time foetal distress occurs more often (Smyth, 1974; Flynn and Kelly, 1976).

We do not yet know much about the effect of the place where birth is conducted, the environment which each society selects for it, whether home, hospital, or a hut in the bush. In those societies where there are marked culture contrasts we might study peasant women having their babies in the village and the same women giving birth in large public hospitals (see Homans, Chapter 9). We might also examine the comparative sociology of midwifery and its forms in different societies and the role of the midwife in relation to other kinds of professionals including the shaman, diviner or obstetrician. We need more careful observation of the ways in which societies prepare women for birth during childhood and adolescence and in pregnancy. Such preparation often forms an important part of puberty rituals. When the rituals are no longer conducted what happens to the preparation? How do women in the West learn about birth? The Jamaican nana visits the expectant mother regularly throughout pregnancy and massages her abdomen to "shape" the baby while talking to and counselling her. In contrast, women attending British antenatal clinics talk of seeing "a sea of faces" and are unlikely to have continuity of care. The antenatal clinic provides reassurance for some mothers but is anxiety-arousing for many others (Kitzinger, 1979, 1981). Cross-cultural studies would also help us to know more about the developing interactive system between mother and neonate from the first moments after delivery, and discover how social institutions either facilitate interaction or make it more difficult (Klaus and Kennell, 1977).

The study of human reproduction requires a multidimensional analysis of the reciprocal effects of society, culture, personality and biology. From the obstetrician's point of view such an analysis shows that the medical model of childbirth accepted as normal in the West is only one among many possible models, and that medical and scientific procedures can be used for non-medical purposes and have a ritual significance far removed from their apparent technical function.

References

Caldeyro-Barcia, R. *et al.* (1960). "Effects of Position Changes on the Intensity and Frequency of Uterine Contractions During Labour". *American Journal of Obstetrics and Gynecology* **80**, 284–286.

Caldeyro-Barcia, R. *et al.* (1980). "Physiological and Psychological Basis for the Modern and Humanized Management of Normal Labour". Paper presented to 6th International Congress of Psychosomatic Medicine in Obstetrics and Gynaecology, September 1980.

Douglas, M. (1970). *Purity and Danger*. Harmondsworth: Penguin.

Dunbar, F. (1946). *Emotions and Bodily Changes*. New York: Columbia University Press.

Flynn, A. and Kelly, J. (1976). "Continuous Fetal Monitoring in the Ambulant Patient in Labour". *British Medical Journal* **2**, 842–843.

Goffman, E. (1971). *Relations in Public*. Harmondsworth: Penguin.

Goffman, E. (1972). *Interaction Ritual*. Harmondsworth: Penguin.

Kaij, L. and Nilsson, A. (1972). "Emotional and Psychotic Illness Following Childbirth". In *Modern Perspectives in Psycho-Obstetrics* (J. C. Howells, ed.). London: Oliver and Boyd.

Kemp, R. S., and Hency, C. (1978). *Child Abuse*. London: Fontana.

Kitzinger, S. (1981). *The Experience of Childbirth*. (4th edn). Harmondsworth: Penguin.

Kitzinger, S. (1972). "Image and Body Fantasy in Preparation for Birth: an Anthropological View". In *The Family* (H. Hirsch, ed.). Basle: Karger.

Kitzinger, S. (1977). *Education and Counselling for Childbirth*. London: Bailliere, Tindall.

Kitzinger, S. (1978a). *Women as Mothers*. London: Fontana.

Kitzinger, S. (1978b). *The Place of Birth*. Oxford: Oxford University Press.

Kitzinger, S. (1979). *The Good Birth Guide*. London: Fontana.

Klauss, M. H. and Kennell, J. H. (1977). *Maternal-Infant Bonding*. St. Louis: C. V. Mosby Company.

Leach, E. (1976). *Culture and Communication*. Cambridge: Cambridge University Press.

Levi-Strauss, C. (1966). *The Savage Mind.* Chicago: University of Chicago Press.
Levi-Strauss, C. (1967). "The Effectiveness of Symbols". In *Structural Anthropology.* New York: Anchor Books.
Richards, M. P. M. (1978). "Possible Effects of Early Separation on Later Development of Children". In *Separation and Special-Care Baby Units, Clinics in Developmental Medicine no. 68.* London: William Heinemann.
Roth, J. A. (1957). "Ritual and Magic in the Control of Contagion". *American Sociological Review* **22,** 310–314.
Smyth, C. N. (1974). "Section of Measurement in Medicine, Biochemics and Human Parturition". *Proceedings of the Royal Society of Medicine* **67,** 189–193.
Stycos, J. M. and Back, J. W. (1964). *The Control of Human Fertility in Jamaica.* New York: Cornell University Press.
Waterman, J. (1952). "The Functions of the Isthmus Uteri". *Caribbean Medical Journal* **14,** 3–4.
World Health Organization (1979). *Traditional Birth Attendants.* Geneva: WHO.

8. Childbirth and Change: a Guatemalan Study

S. COSMINSKY

As a life crisis, birth is not only a universal biological event, but also a culturally patterned process. Various rituals and symbols mark the transition from one phase of life to another for both mother and child. These birth practices are based on certain conceptions about the body and reflect values and themes of the culture. In many societies, a specialist or midwife is a pivotal figure in the birth system and serves as both a medical and a ritual specialist. The role of the midwife and many traditional birth-related practices are being influenced and changed in a variety of ways, especially through the spread of Western medicine, both through directed changes, such as midwifery training pro-grammes, and undirected changes, as through radio advertisements.

This chapter will discuss the beliefs and practices surrounding child-birth in two areas of Guatemala, a highland village and a lowland plantation, and the changes that are occurring in them under the impact of Western medicine. As in many parts of the world, birth is a heavily ritualized process. Viewing ritual as a symbolic code communicating certain aspects of ideology and social structure (Douglas, 1966; Firth, 1973; Turner, 1967), some of the rituals and practices will be analysed in terms of the underlying values and social relationships that they symbolize.

Research Setting

Data was collected through participant observation and interviewing in the community of Chuchexic, a rural district or *aldea* of the town of Santa Lucia Utatlán in the western highlands of Guatemala, and the surrounding hamlets, and on a lowland sugar and coffee *finca* (plantation), Finca San Felipe (a pseudonym) located on the Pacific lowlands of Guatemala.[1] Interviews and observations were with midwives and medical personnel conducting midwifery training programmes, as well as with mothers.

Chuchexic and its surrounding hamlets have a population of approximately 1600 and the whole town or *municipio* of Santa Lucia has a population of 7742 (1973 census). Approximately 96% of the inhabitants of Chuchexic are Quiché-speaking Mayan Indians; the rest are Ladinos.[2] The Indians are primarily subsistence farmers cultivating maize as the staple crop. They supplement their incomes by growing wheat as a cash crop and engaging in wage labour, especially on coastal plantations. The Ladinos are landowners, entrepreneurs, or wage labourers. The Indians live mainly in dispersed households in the rural *aldeas*, whereas the Ladinos mostly live in the town centre. The majority of Indians are Catholic. However, they are split into two groups: one is a reformed Catholicism which centres around the Catholic Action movement and the other is a syncretic form based on sixteenth century Catholicism and Mayan Indian influences. This latter includes the use of the Mayan ritual calendar and shamans, worship of *El Mundo*, the essence or spirit of the earth, and *Aire*, the air, combined with the worship of God, Jesus, Mary, and the Saints. There is also a handful of Protestant or Evangelical converts.

Finca San Felipe is a coffee and sugar plantation with a population of about 690. The adults and older children are wage labourers as well as landless agriculturalists. Men work for cash most of the year, in sugar or coffee production, and women and older children work seasonally at picking coffee and drying sugar cane. The entire family participates in the cultivation of corn and beans on small plots of land provided by the finca owner.

The finca population is of mixed heritage, consisting mainly of second or third generation Indian migrants from different towns in the Western highlands. Approximately two-thirds of the population classify themselves as Indians, the remainder as Ladinos, who originally came from the nearby coastal towns. Many of the Indians are "ladinoized"—i.e. speak Spanish and wear Western dress. Only a few older people still speak Quiché or one of the Indian languages, but many still wear the

Indian skirt (*corte*) and retain various Indian cultural traits, including certain birth and curing practices.

In both locations, over 90% of the births take place at home, attended by a local indigenous or "empirical" midwife. There are several midwives in Chuchexic, but only one at present on the finca. A few women give birth in the hospital, those from Chuchexic going to the departmental capital of Sololá, and those from the finca going to Retalhuleu, but these are usually either for complications, for sterilization, or they are women of higher socio-economic status. There is a Catholic mission clinic in Chuchexic run by nuns, at least one of whom is a nurse-midwife. They run a prenatal clinic and they have given a midwifery training course (Cosminsky, 1978). They also assist in cases of complications and drive emergencies to the hospital in Sololá.

The midwives represent varying degrees of traditionalism, acculturation and Western training, ranging from a traditional Mayan midwife with no Western training to those, both Indian and Ladino, who have attended a midwifery training course and received an official licence (Cosminsky, 1977, n.d.). Despite these differences between Ladino and Indian contexts and the lowland and highland environments, many basic concepts and practices concerning childbirth are shared. These concepts include: (a) the midwife as a ritual, as well as obstetrical specialist, (b) the location and movement of organs, (c) the hot-cold theory, and (d) the influence of emotions and social relations on the body. Differences will be indicated only when they are meaningful to this study.

The Midwife

The indigenous Mayan midwife is regarded as an obstetrical and ritual specialist (Paul, 1975). She is called an *iyom* or *ilonel* in Quiché and *comadrona* in Spanish. The traditional path of recruitment is through supernatural calling. This destiny or *mandado* is revealed in various ways, such as through birth signs and omens, dreams, illness and finding strange objects (shells, scissors, special shaped stones and mirrors). The dreams and signs are interpreted by a diviner or shaman as signifying her destiny as a midwife, and the objects are considered messages sent by the supernatural (God or the spirits). One midwife had found a red and white mirror when she was young, in which she saw the face of a white-haired woman. This was interpreted as being Santa Ana, the patronness of childbirth, and the red was said to symbolize the fire of the sweatbath. If a person does not follow one's calling, she shall suffer supernatural sanctions in the form of illness or death either to herself or members of her family (Cosminsky, n.d.).

Even midwives who do not subscribe to the belief of the supernatural or divine recruitment, such as the Ladino midwives, believe they receive supernatural assistance. They pray to God, to the spirits of the dead midwives (*Comadronas invisibles*), Mary and Saint Ann for the protection of their clients and for assistance. According to the midwives, these spirits tell them if the birth is normal or not, how to massage, what to do if the baby is not in a correct position and what herbs and medicines to use. During a birth, they are accompanied by these spirits.

As part of the process of becoming a midwife, she may have repetitive dreams, such as having babies in her arms and lap, which are interpreted by a shaman as being a sign of her calling. She continues to have special dreams throughout her practice. One midwife said that if she dreams that a man arrives and leaves money in her hand, a boy will be born, and if she finds a shawl or napkin, a girl will be born. Another midwife said she dreams that she is hurrying on a road out of breath, which portends an imminent birth.

Bodily movements, such as twitches or tremblings are also felt. Some midwives said they feel a movement, like air, in the hand or some other part of the body when someone is going to come to call for a birth. If it's in the left hand, the birth will be delayed, and if the right, it will be quick. These bodily manifestations, such as dreams, twitches, and sickness, are regarded as messages from God or the spirits. Supernatural forces are constantly manifested throughout the midwife's body. The body is sacred and is not separated by a boundary from the moral, social, and supernatural context, but is constantly permeated by these influences.

These signs validate the midwife's status as a ritual specialist. She can interpret various signs and omens and mediate between her client and the spiritual world for a safe birth. The supernatural validation also may increase her own confidence and consequently her patient's, and help allay anxieties about birth. In addition to the claim of a supernatural source of knowledge, several of the midwives had been apprenticed to other midwives.

The midwife both in Santa Lucia and on Finca San Felipe is usually an older woman (40 years of age or older) with much prestige and highly respected for her skills, which may be both obstetrical and ritual. In fact, in Santa Lucia, at least four midwives were over 70 years old. Respect is manifested in forms of deference, such as terms of address, kissing of the hand, formalized requests for her aid, godparent relationships and gifts of food and drink. There is also a special bond of respect between the midwife and the children whom she has delivered, who greet her with bowed head and kiss her hand.

Several of the traditional midwives have had training courses given by the Public Health Ministry. The courses were given in Spanish in the departmental capital with an interpreter to translate into Quiché. The success of these programmes and the communication problems involved remain to be evaluated. The training, whether in 1952, the year one of the midwives in Santa Lucia took the course or in 1978, stressed the same things: the importance of asepsis and washing the hands, disinfecting the instruments, the use of the horizontal delivery position, the limitations of the midwife and the recognition of complications which she should refer to the nearest doctor or hospital. Most of the traditional practices were condemned, including the use of herbs, the sweatbath and the kneeling or squatting delivery position (Cosminsky, 1978). The nurses in the mission clinic in Chuchexic have offered a course for new midwives (whereas the public health training course is mainly for already practicing midwives). The official licence and training is offered as an alternative to the divine mandate, opening up the role to others who want to practice. It also marks the increasing secularization of the role. The acquisition of Western medical training and a licence raises one's status, especially if added to one's supernatural mandate. The licence seems to be more important for some of the younger mothers, who mentioned they chose one midwife over another because the former had her licence. It is not clear, however, to what extent the licence alone without supernatural validation confers status to a midwife.

The midwife provides antenatal care, management of labour, and postnatal care, for which she usually charges a $5 or $6 fee. The practices associated with each of these stages will now be described.

Antenatal Care

Antenatal care begins when the mother-in-law or husband requests the midwife to visit the patient, usually between the fifth and seventh month, earlier if it is a primipara. Among the Mayans, the request is made in a formal ritualized language, presenting a gift of food for the midwife and 10¢ or 25¢ for candles and incense for Saint Ann and other saints and spirits to bless the client. The midwife visits and examines the client every 20 or 30 days during the early months and every week during the last month. Before each visit, the traditional midwife prays and burns incense in front of the sweatbath. She asks for help from

God, the spirits of orphans, widows, doctors and midwives, and thanks *El Mundo*, the spirit of the Earth, *Aire*, the spirit of the wind, and Santa Ana, San Augustin and Santa Christina, all of whom aid her in making the patient's delivery successful. At the house of her client, she says an "Our Father", and "In the name of the Father, the Son and the Holy Ghost", making the sign of the cross. One of the Protestant Ladina midwives also stresses the importance of prayer. "I have to help a person because God helps me. I don't believe in anyone, only my God, no doctor, because God is my doctor . . ."

The midwife first looks for bodily changes that signify pregnancy, including the colour of the nipples, the size and shape of the breast, and the swelling and height of the abdomen. One midwife said she can also tell by the woman's eyes, which have an empty (*huero*) or different look. The most important aspects of prenatal care are the examination for the foetal position, palpation and massage of the abdominal area. The midwife gently but firmly massages the abdominal area, moving her hands in opposite directions across the abdomen and along the sides. The massage is believed to help promote an easier birth. Sometimes she also massages the calves and thighs, which is supposed to prevent cramps or problems with the legs. It is believed that the foetus should be in an upright position until the last month, when it turns around. During the examination, she attempts to manipulate the foetus by external version if she feels the baby is not in a correct position. She also estimates when the baby is due. Some midwives say that they can tell whether the baby will be a boy or girl, depending on its position to the right or left side, the height of the abdomen and the pigmentation markings on the mother's face. If the woman gets dark markings on her face, which are considered to be caused by the strength of the baby's blood, the baby will be a boy. There is no internal examination nor listening to the baby's heartbeat.

Women continue working their daily chores throughout pregnancy. It is believed that if she exercises and works, the baby will not be too large, whereas if the mother sleeps too much, the baby may grow too big and cause a difficult delivery. However, she must take care while washing clothes and she should not lift heavy objects. She should not pass over a lasso or sew with a long thread, or the baby will be born with the cord over its neck.

Special care should be taken by the mother during pregnancy, since the woman and foetus are in a physically and spiritually weak state, and thus more susceptible to illness and evil forces. One of the most profound influences on the body is believed to be the degree of "hot" or "cold". As in many parts of Spanish America, foods, herbs, medicines, illnesses and bodily states are classified into categories of hot and cold. These are regarded as innate qualities of substances, often judged by the effect they have on the body or from exposure to sun, water, or physical temperature. A healthy body is one which is in balance; illness is due to excess of hot or cold within the body. Treatment is based on a principle of opposition (Cosminsky, 1975).

A pregnant woman is considered to be in a very hot state, partially because of the accumulated blood in her body. Blood is classified as hot. Therefore, care must be taken to avoid certain foods or medicines that might cause an excess of either quality, harming either her or the foetus. Her excess heat makes her vulnerable to attacks of cold, and too great a contrast, as well as too much of one quality, is considered dangerous. Very cold foods include beans, pork, avocados, certain greens, sodas (Coca Cola, Fanta) and sometimes includes eggs. One midwife said that if a pregnant woman eats eggs or "cold" greens, she would swell from *aire* (air or gas). Other midwives said that the restrictions really depend on the health of the mother and that prenatally, she can eat everything unless she is sick. For example, if a woman has colic or *aire*, which are cold illnesses, she should not eat greens, eggs, or beans since these cold foods will make her worse. She should eat and drink items considered as neutral or "hot", but also avoid very hot substances such as chilli. The midwives generally tell their clients they should eat "alimentos", which are locally defined as nourishing foods (Cosminsky, 1975), but also support the belief they should not eat very cold foods, especially if they have a cold illness. Other food proscriptions have a metaphorical or sympathetic basis, such as restrictions against eating "twinned" fruits, like the *chayote* (Sechium edule), to avoid having twins, or rabbit meat, to avoid having multiple births. There is a wide variation concerning the extent to which the restrictions are followed and they are more relevant if the mother is ill. Many of these restrictions remain ideal rules and are not actually followed by everyone. Dietary restrictions are emphasized more in the postpartum period.

Because poor nutritional status is a common problem among pregnant and lactating women (McGuire, 1976),[3] these dietary restrictions are attacked in the midwifery training programmes and midwives are told that the patient could and should eat everything. The programmes, however, could utilize the accepted practices and add foods that fit into the belief system, e.g. chicken soup and greens classified as hot, rather than try to change the beliefs. Furthermore, the principle of neutralization can be used as an accommodation, that is, mixing a cold food or medicine with a hot one or vice versa to make it more acceptable

(Harwood, 1971). The medical personnel should determine the relevancy of the hot-cold classification. Treatment and advice will be more likely if it is communicated within the midwives and mothers' tradition and with respect for such beliefs.

Physical temperature is also considered critical in maintaining a hot-cold equilibrium state. A pregnant woman should not bathe in cold water late in the day or too often in one day, or else the baby will be born with a cold, or the mother might have pains. They also say that going in the river may cause knots in the legs, leg cramps, or rheumatism, and cold water may cause the mother to swell. The woman should also be careful when washing her hair that she does not get cold. This problem is more critical on the finca, where women wash themselves in the river and put their legs in the water when washing clothes, whereas in Santa Lucia, they usually bathe in the sweathbath and kneel on the riverbank or rocks when they wash clothes in the river.

People report having pregnancy cravings. If these are not satisfied, the child might be miscarried. Several mothers retroactively attributed the cause of their miscarriages to such unfulfilled cravings. Cravings are considered desires of the foetus and are usually for fruit or special meats, earth, salt, or special clay tablets called "Pan de Señor". Nevertheless, the midwives say that the pregnant woman should not eat salt or earth, since these will "cut the blood" and make the woman swell (cause edema). Earth eating, however, does seem to be a relatively common practice according to the midwives, although only a specific type of earth called *tashkal* is eaten. Since too much salt does cause water retention and edema, and the earth may contain parasites, this restriction is a beneficial one.

A pregnant woman must avoid exposure to eclipses, which is believed to cause cleft palate, harelip, other infant deformities or stillbirths. On the finca some anacephalic stillbirths were attributed to the mothers' exposure to an eclipse. It is believed that an eclipse results when the sun or moon is "eaten" and that a part of the foetus will similarly be eaten. For prevention, Mayan women are supposed to wear a piece of metal or iron nails in the form of a cross, or a red cloth around the stomach (Saquic, 1973, p. 101).

Although a pregnant woman is in a weak and vulnerable state, she is also a source of danger to others. Because of her heated state she can give the "evil eye" to infants and young animals (Cosminsky, 1976). In most cases, the evil eye is unintentional.

Children are highly valued and are a primary means of status and respect. According to some of the midwives, sterility may be caused by a "cold womb" which consequently does not receive the semen.

One treatment is to warm the womb in the sweatbath and administer "hot" herbal teas. However, if the sterility is caused by God, the midwife cannot cure it.

Strong emotions, such as anger, fright and sadness can cause illness under ordinary circumstances, and should be particularly avoided during pregnancy and the postnatal period. Several types of complications were attributed by the midwives to the mother having suffered "anger" (*enojos* or *colera*). These problems included premature birth, miscarriage, stillbirths, retained placenta, cold or insufficient milk and a sickly baby. One midwife attributed her own sickly childhood and life to fright (*susto*) her mother had suffered during an earthquake while pregnant with her. Another woman said her baby was weak and sickly because of the fright and sadness she suffered from her father-in-law's death. He was run over by a car when she was three months pregnant. Other causes involve conflicts or beatings by a drunk or aggressive husband, which either cause the foetus to have fright (*susto*) and be stillborn, miscarried, or born prematurely (Cosminsky, 1977).

Emotions and the social relations they stem from can influence the body at any time. Anger is not supposed to be expressed openly. Excess bile is thought to be produced by anger and unless the emotion is resolved body functioning will be impaired. When a pregnant woman is frightened or angry she should go to the midwife for herbal teas with "hot" or "cold" properties, and be massaged to restore the body's equilibrium. Douglas has suggested that controlling the body is an expression of social control (1973, p. 70). In this case, the woman herself is to blame for being angry and endangering her unborn child, not her husband for abusing her. Because the unborn child is endangered by the mother's anger and fright—by her lack of self-control—the woman is socially subordinated to her husband who may lose self-control through drunkenness with relative impunity. These cultural definitions enlist the midwife as an unwitting agent of social control. By working to overcome the risk caused by a woman's emotions she acquiesces to the prevailing definitions of social roles. Not only is an imbalance of emotions and social relations expressed in definitions of dangerous body states, but the crisis of a state such as threatened miscarriage is a stimulus for restoring normal social relations (Manning and Fabrega, 1973, p. 269).

Management of Labour and Delivery

When labour begins, the midwife is summoned. Delivery takes place in the mother's home. The midwife says a prayer when she arrives, palpates the woman's abdomen, examines the position of the baby, and looks for the signs of imminent birth. These are the breaking of the sac, the intensity and frequency of contractions, the position of the baby's head, and the heat, flushing and sweating of the woman. Massaging may be done during labour if the woman is having much pain. This takes the form of downwards movement on the dorsal and frontal sides. According to the nurses in the clinic in Chuchexic, the midwives do not distinguish the different stages of labour and have the woman push too early.

The woman usually delivers in a kneeling position, with the midwife catching the baby from behind. Sometimes she may squat and hold on to a rope. If the husband is present, he is expected to help by holding and supporting the woman, a duty that is intended to teach him what women have to suffer through. The mother or mother-in-law or other female relatives may also be present. The midwifery training courses stress the horizontal (lithotomy or supine) delivery position, as based on American and European obstetrical practices, and discourage the traditional one. In one course, the trainees were told not to use the traditional position because the baby might hit its head on the floor possibly causing brain damage. The probability of this occurring should be questioned.

The manual for training midwives issued by the Guatemalan Ministry of Public Health advises the midwife to arrange the mother in a semi-sitting or physiological position that is most in agreement with the cultural patterns. However, when the dilation is complete, ask the woman to bend her legs, with feet resting on the bed, grasping her ankles, and to push softly. This is accompanied by a picture of a woman lying on her back with her shoulders slightly raised by a pillow, knees bent and feet on the bed—thus reinforcing the idea that the horizontal position is best. The use of the supine position has been recently questioned (Haire, 1972). Although it is easier for the obstetrician or midwife to see, it may be more difficult for the mother and child because it is against gravity and may promote interference. (For a more detailed discussion: cf. Cosminsky, 1977). Care should be taken in the programmes not to eliminate a beneficial practice in favour of one which may be less advantageous and even potentially harmful.

The midwife may also administer remedies—herbal teas if the labour is difficult or delayed. These teas include the root of the *acuzena* (Lilium longiflorum), or *kispar* (Petiveria allionacea), or *pimpinela* (Poterium sanguisorba) mixed with clove and cinnamon. The midwife on the finca also adds oregano, or nine leaves of *Flor de Pascuas* (poinsettias), nine avocado leaves, and 20 drops of *esencia maravillosa*, a liquid made from alcohol and extracts of several herbs sold in the pharmacies. All these herbs are classified as "hot" ones. According to Saquic (1973, p. 10) the Indians in Santa Lucia attribute difficult births to the misbehaviour of the wife, who has to confess. She is given a candle and asks the pardon of God. If this does not help, she is given a drink of oil or yolk of one or two eggs. If she still has trouble, the midwife tells the husband to take off a sandal or shoe and hit the woman three times with it on her back saying that she is forgiven for whatever bad she has done.

The umbilical cord is usually not cut until after the placenta is expelled. If the cord is cut before, it is believed that the child might die, and the placenta might rise up in the woman's body and cause her to choke. If the placenta is retained and the cord must be cut, it is tied to the woman's leg so it will not rise, until she is taken to the nearest doctor or hospital. Some midwives give the woman a little bit of cooking oil to drink which is to help the placenta slide out. Others put the woman's braid or two fingers in her mouth to make her gag and cause contractions to expel the delayed placenta. The body is perceived as a tube in which organs can be displaced or move up and down.

The placenta is thought to have a special relationship to the child and can affect its future. Consequently, proper disposal is necessary. In both Santa Lucia and on the finca, the placenta is burned and the ashes buried. Care must be taken so that dogs will not unearth it, as this will harm the child. Proper disposal is supposed to assure that the person will not wander from his village when an adult.

The courses for traditional midwives teach that one can cut the cord before the placenta is expelled. However, if the cord is cut before it stops pulsing, crucial blood is cut off from the baby, and thus the traditional practice is of some benefit. Medical personnel, however, feel that the midwives wait too long to cut the cord.

Some of the traditional methods for cutting and dressing the cord, such as cauterizing the cord with a candle flame or hot blade have been criticized by medical personnel, who teach the midwives to disinfect the scissors and use alcohol on the cord. Since cauterizing the cord also leaves it sterile, there is no reason why it should be condemned. One nurse said that the candle wax might be dirty, and that's why the practice was harmful. Some midwives have combined the practices, first cauterizing the cord and then using the alcohol and mertiolate (Cosminsky, 1977).

The cord is examined for various signs, which the midwife, as a ritual specialist, has the knowledge and power to interpret. The number of lumps or markings symbolize how many children the woman will have. Round lumps signify girls and long ones males. The distance between

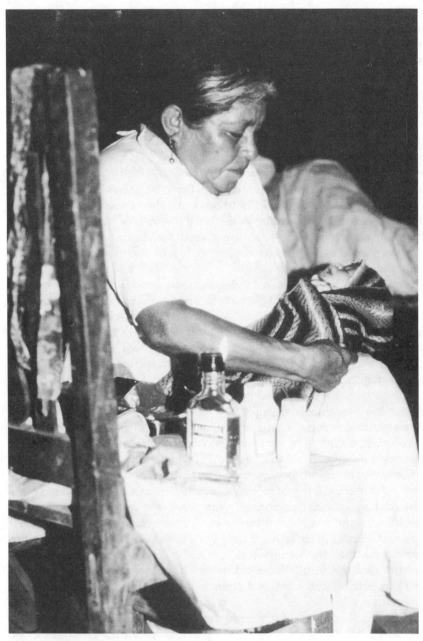

Fig. 1. Guatemalan traditional midwife with swaddled newborn child. Beside her is the candle used to cauterize the end of the umbilical cord and alcohol to dress it.

the markings indicates the birth interval. For example, if the marks are two fingers apart, the interval will be two years. If the cord is short or smooth the mother will not have any more children. If a baby is born in a sac or with a caul, the child may become a transforming witch or *characotel* unless it is removed properly from behind and then burned. Pieces of the sac on the baby indicate certain types of predestined birth, including that of a midwife (Paul, 1975, reports similar beliefs in San Pedro la Laguna). The degree to which these beliefs are held vary among the midwives and mothers. Some maintain certain ones while doubting or being sceptical of others. One midwife said that the pieces of the veil or sac are put there by the midwife herself. With more Western training and less belief in the supernatural power and destiny of the midwife, one can expect a decline in the persistence of these signs and omens, and thus attenuation in this aspect of the ritual role of the midwife.

On the finca, the midwife said that the stump of the cord should be put in a covered jar and saved after it falls off. If the baby is a male, sometimes the cord is put in a tree, so that he will be able to climb when he gets older; if a female, it is put under the hearth so she will do her household duties.

After the birth, the midwife on the finca washes the blood-stained clothes of the mother in the river. This was part of the traditional role of the midwife in some areas of Guatemala. The finca midwife said that she now washes the clothes only if the woman has no other female relatives to help her, because she feels sorry for her. In one of the observed review classes for midwives, the nurse told the midwives not to wash the clothes. She said that the *only* thing the midwife should do is assist with the birth. She should not wash clothes, nor help prepare meals (as some midwives do), nor give medicine. These should not be part of the midwives' duties. If she does such chores, she should charge extra. Some of the nurses complained that untrained midwives charge less and also wash the clothes, thus undercutting them. The nurse defined the midwife's role according to the Western biomedical system as a strictly obstetrical one, but the traditional role is an expanded role, part of a support system that includes social, ritual and psychological components.

Postpartum Care

In Santa Lucia, the postpartum confinement period is 20 days. The 20-day period is equal to one month of the ancient Mayan ritual calendar.

Although the mother can work after 20 days, she should not have sexual relations for 40 days following the birth. This *cuarentena* probably derives from Spanish influence (Foster, 1960, p. 5). On Finca San Felipe, the confinement period is eight days, during which the woman must rest. In each case, the actual number of days and activities of the woman varies according to her physical and nutritional condition, the number of female relatives to assist her and her socio-economic status. The midwife visits the mother every few days during this confinement period to examine and change the dressing on the cord of the baby and to massage the mother. Usually warmed cooking oil or olive oil, or a commercial preparation such as Pomada Valencia is used. Medicated plaster, such as Hazel Menthol may be applied afterwards.

The body is perceived as a tube in which the various parts (organs, veins, bones etc.) may become displaced and lead to illness or complications. The massage is said to return the uterus to its proper place and size and relieve postpartum pains. Fallen uterus is considered by the midwives to be the most common postpartum problem. Some of the midwives also massage the legs, downwards from the thighs and upwards from the calves, for "distended nerves" which can cause pains in the mother's legs and to prevent problems with the veins. The bones of the birth canal are believed to open when the child is born. In order to close the bones, as well as to keep the womb in place, an abdominal binder is then tied below the navel, pushing the abdomen upwards. The physical contact and focus of attention involved in these practices also provides emotional and social support to the mother.

Medical personnel have expressed concern about the massaging being too hard and thus dangerous. They have also discouraged the use of the binder in the hospitals and the training programmes. An understanding of the way these practices are linked to perceptions of the body, as mentioned above, and of their possible beneficial effects (Harrison, 1977) might enable them to adapt the practices in a more compatible manner and thus be more effective. For example, gentle massage might be suggested rather than trying to persuade midwives to give up their practice of massage. The abdominal binder could still be used, but not tied too tightly, and be phrased in terms compatible with the midwives' beliefs.

The mother is in a cold state after the birth and must take proper precautions. Certain dietary restrictions are advised during the confinement period, the most common one being the avoidance of "cold" foods, similar to the restriction during pregnancy. However, they seem to be regarded as more important postnatally because they are thought to cut the mother's milk or make it cold and consequently make the nursing baby ill. Special foods are recommended such as chicken soup, bananas and *atole* (a maize gruel), and "hot" foods (but not too hot like chilli). Relatives, godparents and neighbours visit the woman during this transitional period and bring these foods which are considered good for giving strength and good for lactation. One midwife, however, said that if the woman or child does not have any illness, she can eat everything. "If she eats *alimentos*, she will have good milk and good health." If the child is sick, however, the mother should avoid eating cold things because they make the child worse. She must only wash in warm water and avoid cold baths and cold water, which will make the milk turn cold and watery. The mother's head should be covered with a scarf for 10–15 days and her shoulders covered with a shawl or sweater to prevent getting *aire* (air) and turning the milk cold. Some women expressed anxiety about hospital deliveries because they said they could not keep their head and shoulders covered the way they thought necessary and that the hospital food was not compatible with dietary restrictions.

The midwife administers herbal teas as remedies for postpartum pains, usually made from a mixture of "hot" herbs, such as *artemisia*, *pimpinela* (Poterium sanguisorba), oregano and white honey. One midwife said she no longer uses herbs since she had the training course, because she was told not to use them. The use of herbs at any state in the birth process is condemned by Western medical personnel, based on the assumption that the midwife is ignorant of the effects of the herbs, and some of them may be effective and therefore dangerous if given too large a dosage. However, since some of these plants may have beneficial effects, investigation and analyses should be made of these herbs. The herbal knowledge is being gradually lost and the newly trained midwives are more familiar with patent medicines instead. The traditional midwives say they learn the herbs through dreams or visions, although they may also learn through apprenticeship with another midwife. The decline in the use of herbs and the loss of this knowledge represents an attenuation of the midwife's role resulting from her attempt to adapt to modern medicine, on which she is becoming increasingly dependent.

The application of heat is emphasized, especially in the postnatal period. This may take the form of a sweatbath, among the Indians in Santa Lucia, a sitz bath (*bajo*) as among the Ladinos, or a herbal bath, as on the finca. The heat is believed to help restore the bodily balance. The midwives say that the bath increases the flow of milk, "lowers" the milk into the breasts, prevents it from becoming "cold", protects the woman from *aire*, eases afterbirth pains and promotes healing.

Traditionally, the woman takes a sweatbath every three or four days, during which she is massaged by the midwife. The sweatbath (Quiché: *tuj*; Spanish: *temascal*) is a small adobe structure located adjacent to the house. Inside, rocks are heated and water thrown on top to make steam. The person sits on a wooden board inside the *temascal*. Branches from the plant *kewuj* (*Corepsis mutica*) are used to beat and drive the steam towards the woman. The sweatbath usually lasts about a half hour. One midwife said she gives the first sweatbath on the third day, but not very hot and only for cleaning, not for a massage. On the eighth day, she takes the sweatbath again, making it hotter and massages the woman. She used to visit every 3 or 4 days, but now does it once a week during the 20-day period. The bath provides ritual as well as physical cleansing, since the blood from the birth is regarded as polluting. It also gives emotional and psychological support to the mother. However, the frequency and use of the sweatbath varies and is declining. One of the traditional Mayan midwives said "the sweatbath is my medicine", whereas others do not use it at all. One midwife takes the woman into the sweatbath but only bathes her. She massages her afterwards inside the house and bathes the child in warm water rather than in the sweatbath. Another midwife said that before she received the Public Health training course, she used to enter the sweatbath, but then she was told not to. When she first visits a pregnant woman now, she explains that she will not go into the sweatbath with the woman. Usually the woman will then take a sweatbath herself before the midwife's visit and the midwife will massage her in the home. One of the Ladino midwives also does not use the sweatbath because it gives her a headache and makes her legs bad, although the mothers want it. She said she is not used to it since it is an Indian rather than a Ladino custom. Instead, she uses a vapour bath in which the woman sits over a basin or bucket of hot water containing several herbs, covers herself and lets the steam enter from below.

The sweatbath has been discouraged by official medical personnel. In one observed review class, the nurse giving the course mentioned that some untrained midwives still used the sweatbath, but she did not believe that anyone in the room used if for their patients. The manner and tone of the statement was mocking and condemnatory. The nurse did not give any explanation at that point of why it should not be used, so I asked. The nurse in turn asked the midwives. One Ladino midwife who had never used it said she had heard about a midwife who had an attack and fainted inside the sweatbath with her patient, and that was why it was dangerous. The nurse then said that the sweating might cause dehydration and thus fainting. Other nurses told me they believed the sweatbath was debilitating and promoted haemorrhaging.

How often such dehydration occurs is unknown. The nurse also said that the person might catch pneumonia from the sharp change in temperature if they go outside after the sweatbath. Ironically, the nurse is expressing agreement with the folk theory of illness causation, which attributes an illness like pneumonia to sharp or extreme contrasts of hot and cold. In actuality, people take great care to stay inside, covered up, after taking a sweatbath. To my knowledge, no studies have been made concerning these supposedly harmful effects of the sweatbath, nor of any possible beneficial effects, such as stimulation of blood circulation, milk flow, relaxing muscles, promotion of healing, preventing infection and easing soreness. The effects depend on the intensity, length and frequency of the sweatbaths, and the condition of the woman. Modifications could be suggested in these ways, rather than complete condemnation. Further research should be done in this area.

On the finca, a herbal bath is given on the third day and the eighth day. Until this bath, the woman is not supposed to do any household activities. The herbs used in the bath are "hot" herbs. These are Santa Maria (*Piper* sp.), *guaruma* (*Cercopia peltata*), *ciguapate* (*Pluchea odorata*) and *siguinai* (*Vernonia* sp.). The herbs are put in a bucket of hot water. A handful of the heated herbs are placed under the woman for her to sit on, some are placed in front of the vaginal area, and some under her feet. The feet are considered vulnerable points of entry for *aire* or wind. The midwife rubs the mother's back and breasts with a handful of the herbs as she is bathing her with the hot water. One of the main functions of the bath is to warm and lower the breast milk. One woman became quite anxious when the bath was delayed because the midwife had been called elsewhere. She was concerned about the condition of her milk and the restrictions on her activity. After she was bathed, the midwife made her squeeze out some of the milk first, saying that the milk would still be cold because the herbs had not yet taken effect.

After the bath, the midwife massages the woman and puts on an abdominal binder. On the finca, the bath is repeated on the eighth day, which marks the end of the midwife's duties and mother's seclusion. In Santa Lucia, the last sweatbath is on the twentieth day, at which time a special ritual feast is held, called *elesan xe ch'at* or "taking out from under the bed" (Saquic, 1973, p. 104).

Elesan Xe Ch'at—A Postpartum Ritual

At the end of the 20-day period of confinement, a ritual celebration and feast are held. Preparations usually begin the previous day and continue

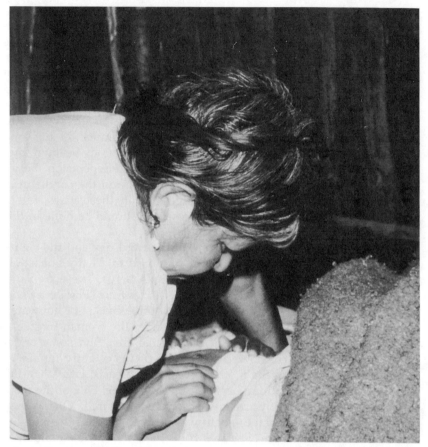

Fig. 2.   Midwife concluding a postnatal massage by applying a binder.

to the day of the celebration. The woman's female relatives (mother, mother-in-law, sisters, sisters-in-law, and some aunts and nieces) help grind the maize, make the *tamalitas* and cook the meat and soup. The male relatives (father, father-in-law, brothers and brothers-in-law) fetch the firewood, cover the floor with pine needles, set up the benches and tables and serve drinks. The couple is responsible for providing the food and drinks.

When the midwife arrives, she goes into the kitchen area and is served some bread and coffee. Later she is given drinks and a serving of the ritual meal. Sometimes the midwife gives the woman a sweatbath first, after which she massages the woman. In one case, the midwife massaged the woman "because she had heat in her stomach". Usually, the abdominal binder is removed at this time.

Previously, all the garbage from whatever the woman ate during the twenty days, such as maize husks from the *tamalitas* and chicken bones, was thrown under the bed. One informant said this is no longer done because it is unhealthy and people know better today. They still observe the ritual cleaning and sweeping, however.

The midwife cleans out the sweatbath, removing the ashes and rubbish that have collected during the postpartum period, and puts them in a basket or bowl, lined with leaves. The husband buries this in the nearby maizefield. While cleaning out the sweatbath, the midwife crosses herself before and after. She lights two candles of wax or tallow on a piece of inverted clay tile, burns some incense and *copal* and sprinkles white roses on the place in the sweatbath where the fire is lit. She offers these in prayer to Santa Ana, patronness of the sweatbath and pregnant women, saying:

> Now they have completed the twenty days, pardon me. I do not have anything to give you, only this bit of candle, this bit of incense. Make use of it, then pardon me. Perhaps I had it in garbage or filth, pardon me, señora, pardon me; it is my blame. You cleansed us. You polished us during the twenty days. You took away all dirtiness. Nothing happened to us. We are all well. The child is with good health and the mother is with good health. Thank you very much.

She also says two "Hail Mary's" and two "Our Fathers", crosses herself and kisses the ground to *El Mundo*, the spirit of the Earth, "who gives us food and life". One midwife who has converted to Protestantism does not make the offerings, but she does clean out the ashes from the sweatbath. The Ladino midwife does not perform the ceremony at all.

The midwife then goes into the room where the woman's bed is, takes off all the bed coverings and blankets and shakes them out. Meanwhile, she crosses herself, prays and says the name of the baby. She dusts off all the boards of the bed with some branches and leaves. She takes the middle board off, and taps the other bedboards with the edge, in the sign of a cross, repeating the name of the newborn baby. She then sweeps out all the pine needles and rubbish from under the bed. This is burned and buried together with the ashes from the sweatbath. Variation exists in the extent to which this ritual is carried out. One midwife reversed the order, cleaning the bed out first and then the sweatbath; another cleaned out the sweatbath, swept under the bed, but did not clean the bed or bedclothes. The Ladino midwife cleans neither the sweatbath, bed, or bedroom, instead, she gives the woman a purgative on the twentieth day.

As suggested in an earlier paper (Cosminsky, 1976), the ritual cleaning of the bed and the sweatbath may be a symbolic acting out of the cleaning referred to in the prayer. The ritual marks the status transition from an "unclean" state to a condition of "cleanliness". As the sweat-bath and its patronness, Santa Ana, have "cleansed" the woman, so does the midwife clean the sweathbath and the bed. Blood (which is regarded as polluting), bodily wastes and left over wastes from food are separated out as dirt. As Douglas (1966) suggests, what is considered "dirt" symbolizes disorder. Elimination of it is an attempt to organize the environment. All this "dirt" is buried together in the fields, into the formlessness of garbage and earth, thus restoring order. Similarly, the ceremony marks the mother's and child's integration into the social order. Saquic, who is originally from Santa Lucia (1973, p. 104), says the ritual symbolizes a new life.

Drinks of rum are then passed around, first to the men, then to the midwife and lastly to the women, who stay in the kitchen. The meal of soup, meat and tamalitas is served, the men eating first, either in the main room or on tables set up in the patio, and the women in the kitchen. The children eat either in the main room or in the kitchen after the men have been served. After the meal, the women send baskets containing food to various relatives, neighbours and godparents, pri-marily people who had visited the woman during the 20-day period and with whom she has reciprocal obligations. The young girls and women carry the food to the various houses.

The midwife may also pierce the ears of a female child on this day. In one observed case, the midwife first rubbed the child's ear to make it numb. She threaded a needle with red thread (possibly because red is used against the evil eye), heated it, and pierced the baby's ears, tying the thread in a loop.

The *elesan ch'at* ceremony marks the end of the midwife's duties and obligations, and the end of the mother's seclusion, which was regarded as the most dangerous period for the mother and child. The joint participation of relatives from both sides of the family emphasizes the importance of the birth in continuing the family lines and cementing the bonds, as well as reinforcing family solidarity. This is also sym-bolized in the exchange of food mentioned above. The woman is re-integrated into her family role and both mother and infant are given social support and recognition of their new status. (Paul and Paul, 1975, describe a similar postnatal bath and ritual carried out on the eighth day among the Zutuhil Maya in San Pedro la Laguna.)

The frequency of this ritual is declining, despite its seeming impor-tance. Several people mentioned that they have not given it or only gave it for some of their children. One person said that the only reason they gave it this time (August, 1974) was because the particular midwife would gossip about them to other people. Although this personality trait was criticized, it served as an effective mechanism of social control. The fear of social pressure indicates that probably the majority of people still regard the ceremony as necessary and critical. This particular family had not had the ceremony for their other two children (despite the fact that the paternal grandfather was a shaman); they had also used a different midwife then. Another person said she would have the midwife clean out the sweatbath and give her some food, but felt they could not afford the ritual meal with the relatives. The celebration is expensive relative to the material wealth of these families. Three people said they used about 40 lb maize, 10 lb meat, potatoes, chayotes and other vegetables, bread, rum, and coffee. Since the price of maize has tripled between 1968 and 1974, the economic factor will probably become increasingly important. However, the ritual's decline also marks a decreasing adherence to and sharing of certain symbols and beliefs associated with the ritual.

Conclusion

The concepts and practices of the indigenous birth system in Guatemala present a sharp contrast to those promoted by Western medicine in the health care facilities, prenatal clinics and midwifery training programmes, which are based on the biomedical model of birth. In this framework, pregnancy is viewed as a disease; it is a physical bodily disturbance and is medicalized. The birth specialist performs a medical or obstetrical role. The body is separated from the self and its social and physical environment. In contrast, the indigenous Mayan view of birth is part of a holistic and personalistic system, involving moral values, social relations and the environment, as well as physical aspects. Furthermore, as Manning and Fabrega have suggested, for the Maya of Chiapas, Mexico, the body is a sacred concept rather than a mechanistic one with a "machine-like instrumentality" (1973, p. 278).

One aspect of this holistic system is the maintaining of the hot-cold balance or equilibrium both within the body and with the environment. This is related to the importance of heat, which seems to be not only related to the hot-cold balance but also to the concept of cleansing of pollution. Heat has semantic associations with blood and fertility, both symbolic of women. Blood is usually considered "hot", although there are varying degrees of hotness. A pregnant woman is considered as being in an unusually hot condition, whereas after delivery, the woman is in a cold state, both from the loss of blood and the expulsion of the baby. Therefore, she needs heat, both with respect to qualitative and physical temperature. As mentioned earlier, she is given "hot" foods and herbal teas, hot postnatal baths or sweatbaths, and avoids cold foods and substances. During the massages, the midwife's hands and the oil she uses are warmed. Heat is nourishing for both the mother and child. Heat, either in the sweatbath or herbal bath, is cleansing and purifying, both physically and spiritually. This is elaborated in the 20-day postpartum ritual where the woman, the bed, the baby and the sweatbath are all cleansed.

Not only must a balance be maintained between the hot and cold states, but also of emotional states and social relations. The centrality of emotions and the equilibrium of social relations, especially within the family, is another aspect of the indigenous holistic model. Medical personnel should be made aware of the importance of emotions in the local belief system, in the management of pregnancy and childbirth, and their influence on the birth process.

The sacred and ritual aspects of the birth process, and the midwife's role, are being attenuated in the process of change (Landy, 1974). The concept of divine mandate is declining and the official licence and training is being offered as an alternative, primarily for younger women. The midwife's role as mediator between her client and the supernatural, including Santa Ana, the spirits of dead midwives, El Mundo, God, Jesus and Mary, is declining. This change can be seen especially in the decreasing practice of the 20-day postpartum ceremony with its prayers, cleaning and ritual meal. The midwife cannot perform certain rituals and interpret signs if she is not supernaturally validated and does not have the power or "call". The decrease in the sacred aspects of the midwife's role and increasing secularization also probably reflects a decrease in the extent to which some of these beliefs and symbols are shared among the client population, as a result of other changes in religion (the Catholic Action movement and Protestantism), in wage labour and in education, as well as from the spread of western medicine.

The midwife plays a role in social control and in maintaining the traditional system. She is a repository of traditional practices and beliefs, some of which she imparts to the mother in the form of advice and dietary and behavioral restrictions, and others which are incorporated into rituals and backed by supernatural sanctions. If a particular ritual is not held and Santa Ana not properly thanked, some misfortune may occur to either the child or mother.

The midwife is an agent of social control also through gossip and other informal sanctions. The woman who said she had held the *elesan xe ch'at* ceremony because the "midwife talks", was not worried about supernatural sanctions but about social pressures. The midwife exerts influence through her higher social status, and works towards maintaining the traditional role of the female and mother (although ironically her role violates many of the general female restrictions, cf. Paul, 1975). Although the midwife may actually increase the anxiety of the mother in this respect, much of her behaviour seems to allay the mother's fears. The midwife's visits, massages, advice, prayers and rituals provide the mother with social and emotional support, all of which can help reduce the anxieties associated with the life crisis of birth. However, the increasing secularization of her role represents a narrowing of her role to little more than an obstetrical one.

The midwife can also be an agent of change. Incorporation of certain practices and medicine, such as the use of alcohol and mertiolate on the umbilical cord, reflects an adaptive change, especially where midwives have added these practices to the beneficial traditional one of cauterizing the cord. At the same time that there is an expansion of the midwife's knowledge concerning aspects of biomedicine, there may be a curtailment of traditional knowledge. She is told in the training programmes not to use herbs, not to use the sweatbath, not to use the traditional delivery position, not to do household duties for the mother, not to massage and not to handle complications, but refer them to the doctor. If they accept this "modern" attenuated role, their knowledge will not be passed on to new midwives.

The general tone is strongly negative toward the traditional practices, condemning them and encouraging the imposition of Western ones. No attempt has been made at accommodating any possible beneficial aspects or of adding the Western practices, rather than substituting them. A number of practices are either positive or innocuous in their benefits and there are some about whose effects very little is known, "although they are prohibited or denounced in carte blanche fashion by the medical establishment" (Harrison, 1977, p. 31). Although programmatic statements have been made concerning the need for health programmes, including midwifery training programmes, to include anthropological concepts and consider the local beliefs, practices, social context and specialists (Kelly, 1956; Verderese and Turnbull, 1975; Cosminsky, 1978), this remains an ideal that has not yet been realized. Such considerations have rarely been incorporated in programmes in Guatemala. There seems to have been little attempt to understand, build on or incorporate these into the training or health programmes, but rather to eradicate them (Harrison, 1977). The birth concepts and practices of the midwives and the client population discussed in this paper are not merely "superstitions" or "problems" to be ignored or eliminated, they are ways people have devised to cope with the crisis of birth and are intimately related to other aspects of the social milieu.

Changes are occurring in the indigenous birth system. Attempts to make both these changes and the training and medical programmes that are promoting them more compatible with the sociocultural framework of the local population would also make for more effective programmes and, hopefully, improved maternal and child health.

Notes

(1) Fieldwork in Santa Lucia was supported in 1968–1969 with a fellowship from the Institute of Nutrition of Central America and Panama (INCAP) and the National Institutes of Health, and in the summer of 1974 through a grant from the Rutgers University Research Council. Fieldwork on Finca San Felipe (pseudonym) has been carried on at different intervals in several trips from 1974–1978, and supported by grants from the Williams-Waterman Foundation, Massachusetts Institute of Technology and the Rutgers University Research Council. I would also like to express my appreciation to Dr Nevin Scrimshaw for his support and assistance and to Dr Lorin Nevling, Jr, of the Field Museum of Chicago for the plant identifications.

(2) The term "Ladino" refers both to descendants of former Spanish or mixed Spanish-Indian ancestry and to people oriented towards Spanish or Western culture in contrast to those oriented towards Indian culture.

(3) A study of dietary intake of a sample of the plantation women showed only eight percent of the pregnant and none of the lactating women were meeting the INCAP recommended dietary levels for calories, protein, riboflavin or niacin levels, 31% of the pregnant women and 12% of the lactating women were below 50% of the recommended protein level whereas none of the non-pregnant and non-lactating women were that low.

References

Cosminsky, S. (1976). "Birth Rituals and Symbolism: A Quiché Maya-Black Carib Comparison". In *Ritual and Symbol in Native Central America* (P. Young and J. Howe, eds). University of Oregon, Anthropological Papers No. 9.

Cosminsky, S. (1977). "Childbirth and Midwifery on a Guatemalan Finca". *Medical Anthropology* **1** (3), 69–104.

Cosminsky, S.. (1978). "Midwifery and Medical Anthropology". In *Modern Medicine and Medical Anthropology in the United States-Mexico Border Population* (B. Velimirovic, ed.). Washington: Pan American Health Organization. Scientific Publ. No. 359.

Cosminsky, S. (n.d.). "Role Adaptation among Indigenous Midwives: A Case Study in a Guatemalan Mayan Community. To be published.

Douglas, M. (1966). *Purity and Danger*. New York: Praeger.

Douglas, M. (1970). *Natural Symbols*. New York: Pantheon Books.

Firth, R. (1973). *Symbols: Public and Private*. Ithaca: Cornell University Press.

Foster, G. (1960). *Culture and Conquest*. Viking Fund Publication in Anthropology No. 27. Chicago: Quadrangle Books.

Harrison, P. (1977). Adiestramiento de Comadronas Tradicionales. Report of Comadrona Section, Maternal-Child Health Study, Health Sector Assessment. Unpublished Draft. Guatemala, Academia de Ciencias.

Harwood, A. (1971). "The Hot-Cold Theory of Disease: Implications for Treatment of Puerto-Rican Patients". *The Journal of the American Medical Association* **216**, 1153–1158.

Kelly, I. (1956). "An Anthropological Approach to Midwifery Training in Mexico". *Journal of Tropical Pediatrics* **1**, 200–205.

Landy, D. (1974). "Role Adaptation: Traditional Curers Under the Impact of Western Medicine". *American Ethnologist* **1**, 103–127.

Manning, P. and Fabrega, H. (1973). "The Experience of Self and Body: Health and Illness in the Chiapas Highlands". In *Phenomenological Sociology* (G. Psathas, ed.), pp. 251–301. New York: John Wiley.

McGuire, J. (1976). A Dietary Survey of Guatemalan Women on the Finca San Luis. Unpublished manuscript.

Ministerio de Salud Publica y Asistencia Social, Guatemala. (1976). *Manual para adiestramiento de comadronas tradicionales*. 3a Revision.

Paul, L. (1975). "Recruitment to a Ritual Role: The Midwife in a Maya Community". *Ethos* **3**, 449–467.

Paul, L. and Paul, B. (1975). "The Maya Midwife as a Sacred Specialist: A Guatemalan Case". *American Ethnologist* **2**, 707–726.

Saquic, R. (1973). "La Mujer Indigena Guatemalteca". *Guatemala Indigena* **8**, 81–116.

Turner, V. (1967). *The Forest of Symbols*. Ithaca: Cornell University Press.

Verderese, M. de Lourdes and Turnbull, L. (1975). *The Traditional Birth Attendant in Maternal and Child Health and Family Planning*. Geneva: WHO. Offset Publication No. 18.

World Health Organization (1979). *Traditional Birth Attendants*. Geneva: WHO. Offset Publication No. 44.

9. Pregnancy and Birth as Rites of Passage for two groups of Women in Britain

H. Homans

Introduction

Pregnancy and birth are widely associated with rituals that transform a woman from the impotence of childlessness to motherhood; from being a young wife to a mature women with the enhanced social status conferred upon mothers in many societies (Van Gennep, 1908; Carlebach, 1966; Ford, 1964; Freedman, 1949; Kitzinger, 1978; Leach, 1976; Paige and Jeffrey, 1973; Saunders, 1954; Pickering, 1974). This chapter looks at the social relations at play in the period of transition, and the perceptions of women undergoing the status transformation. Much of the literature, often from small scale agricultural societies, assumes that the women undergoing rituals of status transformation are socially homogeneous. But in many societies, especially in pluralistic industrial societies, the transition experiences women have, and their responses to them, depend to some extent on their social class and ethnic origins. Pregnancy and birth rituals may have a particular role in reproducing values held by the politically dominant groups, encouraging a particular sexual and social division of labour.[1]

Methods

The chapter is based on interviews in a British Midlands industrial city in 1977 with 39 immigrant women from South Asia (the Indian subcontinent),[2] and 39 British women. They were first interviewed during their initial visit to a consultant antenatal clinic.[3] Twenty-six of the Asian and 26 of the British women were given a second long, structured interview during their eighth month of pregnancy, in their home, with an interpreter if necessary. Because the majority of Asian women in the sample had migrated from rural Punjab (73%), I will focus on the Punjab as a sociocultural homeland. Seventeen (66%) Asian women had lived in the city under study for less than five years.[4] Seventeen (65%) of the Asian women had moved to the city on marriage. By contrast, 22 (85%) of the British women had lived in the city all their life. Eleven (42%) Asian women were living in an extended family at the time of the research and three (12%) of the British women were. Seventeen (66%) Asian women and 24 (92%) British women had relatives living in the same city; so although the Asian women were more likely to be living with relatives, they were less likely to have relatives in the same city.

The Asian women came from four different religions: 13 (50%) women were Sikh; eight (31%) women were Hindu; four (15%) women were Muslim; and one woman was Christian (of the untouchable caste—see Note 6). The British women were either Church of England (73%) or Roman Catholic (27%).

For British women, education and social class position were closely correlated. Sixteen (62%) of the women had left school before age 16 and ten (38%) women had received education beyond the age of 16. Education for the Asian women was not such a useful index of social status, as the land-owning Punjabi Sikhs do not place much value on the education of their daughters, while the Hindu business families considered education to be important in raising their daughter's status.

Status of Women as Reproducers

The social status of pregnant women depends upon the value a society places on motherhood and children. In this comparison, although North India and Britain have different economies, plough agriculture in the former and industrial production in the latter, in both societies women have only a marginal role in production outside the home.[5] Most of the Punjabi women were from the *Jat* caste of land-owning farmers, and most had not worked outside the home.[6] Two were from agricultural labourer families, and one said she had been a seasonal agricultural worker. Women primarily cooked, gave services to male workers and other family members, and produced children. Male children who would contribute to the family as future workers were particularly wanted.

Childless women are therefore accorded low status and barren wives are stigmatized. They can be returned to their family of origin, and are often accused of causing miscarriages by possessing evil spirits. Family planning programmes have not been popular, and pregnancy in a married woman, even a poor or low caste woman, makes her an object of envy (c.f. Marshall, 1973; Mamdani, 1972).

Women who have borne sons have a higher status than those who have only daughters. Sons farm, and bring a wife into the family to help with domestic labour and produce more sons. Daughters on the other hand are a financial liability. They marry and move to the home of their husband taking with them a substantial dowry. A traditional Punjabi saying teaches that "a daughter is a guest in her parents' house", and "bringing up a daughter is like manuring and watering a plant in someone else's courtyard" (Morpeth, 1979).

In Britain, the status of women as mothers is more ambiguous (cf. Myrdal and Klein, 1956; Beechey, 1977). Women have become increasingly involved in paid employment outside the home since the Second World War (Land, 1976, p. 118). Women have more control over their fertility and average family size has decreased. Thus women in Britain may have a self-identity which is not necessarily one of motherhood. However this is not to suggest that women unilaterally derive satisfaction from work outside the home, for this would be to ignore the class differences between women which to a large extent determine the kind of employment they have. What it does suggest is that women do not automatically consider motherhood to be their primary adult role.

Moreover, motherhood may be welcomed by some in a woman's reference group but not by the whole society. For example, grandparents and husbands show sympathy and respect by performing domestic tasks willingly which they would not otherwise do (Homans, 1980, pp. 517–529).

To achieve enhanced status the pregnant woman in Britain must fulfil certain conditions. One condition is that the birth is legitimate and the woman is married. Women who are not married are referred to as if they were married when they attend the antenatal clinic. Hostility is often expressed to women who conceive outside marriage, both by doctors and others. Other categories of women who may be seen to "deviate" from cultural norms are low-class women and immigrants. The controversy which has surrounded these groups has been expressed by Gill *et al.* (1970), McIntyre (1975, 1977), Pearson (1973) and Weeks (1976) in the case of illegitimacy; McKinlay (1970, 1972), Milio (1975), Smith (1970), Stevens (1971) and Sir Keith Joseph (1974) with regard to low-class women and their unwillingness to control their reproduction or use maternal health services. Galloway (1965, 1968) and Powell (1969) have been the most vehement in their attack upon what they consider to be the inordinately high rates of reproduction amongst "coloured" immigrants.

Turning to Asian women's views of their own fertility, one Punjabi woman in the sample spoke of a friend who was so desperate to become pregnant that she experienced a "phantom pregnancy".

> She [the friend] was married about ten years I think and she didn't have any babies at all. And about a year ago, me Mum told me she was pregnant. And I keep on thinking about her you know, that it's good and all that. So I asked me Mum when it was nine months and all that "What's she had?". But the doctor told her that she didn't have anything at all. But she used to say that she's feeling kicking and she's feeling sick and all that you know. After ten months she didn't have anything and they gave her pills to clean her. . . . She really wanted it, she was really happy for nine months. I think it was just imagination with her.

This account suggests the continuing importance of motherhood to Asian women residing in Britain.

Most of the British women also placed importance on becoming a mother and three out of the five British women who had not given birth in the first four years of marriage had been treated for infertility. One of the other women had been waiting for an appointment to see the gynaecologist when she conceived. Pregnancy for these women meant something they had been looking forward to for a long time. As one woman said, "I can't wait for it. I've waited nine years for this" (British working-class woman, two previous miscarriages).

Although the women in this study did not view childlessness as a welcome condition, it would be unwise to assume their views are universally held. Recently the idea of voluntary childlessness has been purported as a viable alternative to motherhood; the slogan "None is fun" was widely espoused by Peck (1973) in America. However, it would appear that this ideology is primarily restricted to white middle-class women. Research in London shows that childlessness is taken more seriously by working-class women who do not have alternative means of self-fulfilment (Newton, 1979).

The Asian and British women studied expected to have a child at some stage in their fertile years, though there were significant differences between the two samples as to when their first child was born. The Asian women, all of whom were married, were far more likely to conceive soon after marriage. Eighty-four percent of the Asian women had given birth before they had been married two years. The married British women, 81% of the British sample, were more likely to wait longer after their marriage before giving birth. Sixty-six per cent of these women gave birth after two or more years of marriage (see Table I). Four (15%) of the British women were not married when they first become pregnant. These figures suggest that there are strong social pressures on Asian women residing in Britain to conceive soon after marriage. Only one of the first-time pregnant Asian women said she had been using contraceptives after marriage. This woman had been educated in Britain and said she came from a "liberal" home.

Mothers and Wage Employment

Although women in Britain can derive status from paid employment as well as motherhood, most women with young children are likely to stay at home to look after them until they are of school age at least. In 1971 less than one-fifth of mothers with children under five years and two-fifths of those with children of primary school age worked either full or part-time, whereas half the mothers with children of secondary school age went to work (Land, 1976, p. 118). One of the reasons women with under school-age children do not work outside the home is the shortage of adequate child care provision. Another reason, however, is the dominant ideology of mothers being individually responsible for their children. This ideology was strongly espoused, for example, by Beveridge in his report on social services (1942). He claims that maternity is "the principle object of marriage" (p. 50), and "in the national interest it is important that the interruption by childbirth should be as complete as possible, the expectant mother should be under no economic pressure to continue work" (p. 49).

In the 1950s Bowlby (1951) stressed the importance of the family as the "correct" socializing agency for the rearing of children. More importantly, he emphasized the exclusive early mother–child relationship as crucial to the future well-being of the child. The physical and psychological development of the child, according to Bowlby, depended on the mother's total care for the child up to school age.

The contradiction between being a "good" mother who stays at home

TABLE I
Time Interval Between Respondents' Marriage and Birth of First Child

Final sample	Asian		British		Total	
	No.	%	No.	%	No.	%
Pregnant and not married	5	19	4	15	4	8
Number of years after marriage woman gave birth						
Same year as marriage	5	19	3	12	8	15
One year after marriage	17	65	5	19	22	42
Two years after marriage	1	4	4	15	5	10
Three years after marriage	2	8	4	15	6	11
Four years after marriage			1	4	1	2
More than five years after marriage[1]	1	4	5	20	6	12
TOTAL	26	100	26	100	52	100

[1] The Asian woman had been temporarily separated from her husband when he migrated to Britain where she joined him after three and a half years.
Three of the British women in this group were treated for infertility and one woman was awaiting an appointment with the gynaecologist when she conceived.

to look after children, at least until school age, and being economically active outside the home, is not easy to resolve. Economic necessity is one determining factor, the extent to which a mother can rely on familial support for child care is another.

The women in this study were asked at the time of their first interview if they were working outside the home. Six of the nine first-time pregnant British women were working, but only one of the nine first-time pregnant Asian women was. The reasons the Asian women gave for not working outside the home were (1) lack of spoken English, (2) not long arrived in this country and (3) their qualifications were not recognized in Britain.

The women were also asked when they were eight months pregnant if they intended to engage in paid employment after the birth of the baby. The responses from both British and Asian women were remarkably similar and fell into four main categories (see Table II). One group of seven (13%) women (four Asian and three British) said they would have to engage in paid employment after the birth of the baby because it was economically necessary.

Without work, one can't manage. Whatever time I find free I do some stitching. I have been stitching from the very beginning. In England I've only worked for five months (outside the home) after my first baby was born, in the canteen, and then again my periods stopped coming—I was going to have another baby. So I worked only for five months. After that the other one followed and I just couldn't work outside the home. (Sikh woman, fifth pregnancy, home worker)[7].

I would like to go back to work. I would have the baby at the nursery as well 'cos they take them from any age. . . . It's just a case of whether I could get a job. The money would help. (British woman, working-class, third pregnancy).

All of the British women who said they needed to work for financial reasons were working-class women.

A second group consisted of eight (13%) women who wanted to work outside the home because they were lonely (three Asian women); interested in careers (three middle-class British women); or just fed up with being a Mum (two working-class British women).

I feel lonely with nothing to do at home. (Educated Hindu woman, first pregnancy).

I'm career-orientated rather than Mother, sort of. Finding great satisfaction in motherhood and just being a wife doesn't interest me—I've got to have some outside interests. (British woman, middle-class, second pregnancy).

TABLE II

Women's Intention to Stay at Home or Engage in Paid Employment after the Birth of the Baby

Final sample	Asian		British		Total	
	No.	%	No.	%	No.	%
Reason for decision						
1. *Will engage in paid employment*						
Economically necessary	4	15	3	11.5	7	13
Social reasons—career, lonely	3	12	5	19	8	15
2. *Do not intend to engage in paid employment*						
No one to look after children	6	23	0	0	6	12
Their duty to stay at home	5	19	8	31	13	25
Husband will not let them	3	12	0	0	3	6
Like it at home	0	0	3	11.5	3	6
Want more children	1	4	2	8	3	6
Had baby because lonely at home	0	0	1	4	1	2
3. *No plans at the moment*	4	15	4	15	8	15
TOTAL	26	100	26	100	52	100

It's good if you work, instead of sitting uselessly at home. (Sikh woman, second pregnancy).

I would love one [a job after this pregnancy]. To be me again, not to be a slave, a machine for everyone. . . . The children don't need you twenty-four hours a day . . . a child needs you most when it's sick, it's ill. (British woman, working-class, fifth pregnancy).

The women in this group felt they needed an identity other than motherhood which they hoped to find in the company of people outside the home.

A third category, containing six of the Asian women living in nuclear families, found they could not work outside the home because there was no one to look after the children.

How can I leave them and work? (Sikh woman, third pregnancy, living in nuclear family).

No. It will be difficult with the children. (Sikh woman, second pregnancy, living in nuclear family).

The largest category, 13 women (25%) (five Asian and eight British) felt it was their duty to stay at home and look after the children, especially until school age.

I don't think you should work really until they go to school. (British middle-class woman, second pregnancy).

I think, let the baby grow for about three years and when the baby's older. (Hindu woman, educated, second pregnancy).

Some women felt particularly uneasy about the prospect of leaving the children in the care of someone else.

I don't feel I can trust anyone else with the children. (British middle-class woman, third pregnancy).

I would like to work. But how can you do it with the children to look after? If I leave them with someone else I don't feel easy. (Hindu woman, sixth pregnancy).

These different responses show the way in which women react to the various ideologies about women as mothers and workers. The first group of women did not see any choice, they had to work to earn money. The second group of women did not particularly identify themselves with the image of mother and wanted to work outside the home in order to gain an independent identity. The third group of women did not have relatives present to help with child-care. This is an important point, for three of the Asian women who said they were going out to work after the birth of the baby were relying on their mother-in-law to look after the baby. In one Punjabi household the mother-in-law was looking after the children of her three daughters-in-law while they went out to work to contribute to the family income. The final group of women illustrates the ideology referred to earlier of the mother being solely responsible for the child for the first few years of its life.

From the women's responses it would appear that it was mainly the British middle-class women who derived status from work outside the home (these women were predominantly teachers who had a more flexible working day than other workers). The lower social class Asian and British women tended to work outside the home because it was economically necessary. This work was in no sense "liberating", nor did it give them high status. Two of the British working-class women considered motherhood gave them a legitimate reason to terminate a boring job.

> I worked at GEC [General Electric Company] right from when I left school till I got pregnant [12 years]. I couldn't stand it you know. I was never happy in my work anyway, it was just one of those jobs I went into you know, because I didn't have any qualifications so. There's not many jobs you can get anyway, and the money was there. (British working-class woman, first pregnancy).

Some women had no choice over whether they worked or not. This was most marked among the Muslim women in the Asian sample who said,

> Our men don't want us to work. They don't like us to go out. (Muslim woman, fourth pregnancy).

The question of whether a woman considers her primary social identity to be that of mother depends greatly on the woman's cultural background, social class position and her relationship with her husband, or male partner.

Management of Pregnancy

In the Punjab most births still take place in the home (Gideon, 1962; Morpeth, 1979). Some traditional midwives (*dais*) have now received formal midwifery training. Ideally, women in the sixth to seventh month of their first pregnancy return to their mother's home. A pregnant woman's behaviour is very much prescribed by older women; especially her mother and her mother-in-law.

The labouring woman is attended by the village *dai*, her mother (or mother-in-law) and possibly her *būa* (father's sister-in-law). Only the very rich, or women having complications in pregnancy, give birth in hospital, where treatment must be paid for. Only four (15%) of the women studied had previously given birth in Asia, and all of these women had a home delivery. Their accounts of the birth were very similar: at home with women they knew and no medical intervention.

Only one Asian woman had been into hospital in India for treatment. She had gone when she was five years old and could not remember much about her visit. Two other women had accompanied relatives to the nearest hospital. One had been with her grandmother when she had her eyes tested, the other woman had visited her younger brother when he was hospitalized. Therefore the Asian women studied had very little experience of hospital care before they migrated to Britain. Their comments about the hospital services in India always referred to the fact that care had to be paid for.

The treatment in the hospital costs money. (Punjabi woman migrated to Britain on marriage, aged 21).

There is a difference as you must know—they [medical staff] look after you better here [Britain] and without money. (Punjabi woman migrated to Britain on marriage, aged 20).

When faced with hospital antenatal care in Britain these women have very little idea of what to expect although they are very grateful that the services are free under the National Health Service. However, the status of pregnant women in Britain is more ambiguous than it is in the Punjab; for pregnancy itself is considered to be potentially pathological by members of the medical profession and therefore requires constant screening and supervision. One possible explanation for the treatment of the pregnant woman in Britain is provided by Oakley. She sees male envy of women's procreative ability being expressed:

in the medical establishment's tendency to assert rigid and authoritarian control over the patterning of pregnancy, labour, and delivery. The pregnant woman is a "patient", a sick person: pregnancy is a pathological process, delivery a clinical procedure complicated by all sorts of difficulties and dangers. To say some-one is ill is one of the most effective ways of robbing them of autonomy and authority (1976, p. 57).

However, to suggest that the neglect of human relations within obstetrics in industrial society today is the result of male envy of women's reproductive capacity is to oversimplify the case grossly. After the Second World War there was considerable concern for the continued reproduction of the population. This anxiety coupled with the publication of the 1958 Perinatal Mortality Survey (Butler and Bonham, 1963), which argues for the medicalization of pregnancy and childbirth through rigorous screening as a means of reducing the mortality rates, has aided the development of clinical medicine and continued male hegemony in the maternal health services. The publication of Government Reports (Guillebaud, 1955; Cranbrook, 1958; Peel, 1970)[8] strengthened the argument for the hospitalization of childbirth and the concomitant concentration of finance in the hospital sector.

Visits to the antenatal clinic often involve long waits, averaging two hours in the clinic studied, and the British women were particularly annoyed by the experience which to them seemed like a production line.[9]

> They see so many there don't they? Oh dear, it's a proper production line there! (British woman, middle-class, second pregnancy).

> I don't like it down the hospital, no, I think it's horrible, well it's like . . . er. . . . You're not an individual, you're just a pack of fat ladies and that's it. You're sort of one in and one out. It's just like a cattle market really. There's no personal—you don't get a personal relationship with your doctor or anything. . . . (British working-class woman, first pregnancy).

The height of de-personalization to some women is the "internal examination" during which they feel reduced "from a person to a pelvic" as Henslin (1971) puts it. Also "an internal examination for a pregnant woman can be both painful and humiliating" (Moyes, 1977). This is what some of the British women interviewed found.

> Mr. X he used to frighten every woman because he'd got very large hands, and everyone was terrified of him. You'd only got to mention X and everybody got the colly wobbles! (British working-class woman, fifth pregnancy).

The Asian women interviewed were so embarrassed by the internal examination they found it difficult to talk about. Their response almost unanimously was that they would prefer to have a woman doctor for this examination.

> I thought always the lady doctor examined you from the inside, because I was examined by a lady the first time, I never thought a man would do it! . . . (Hindu woman, first pregnancy).

One feels shy in any case, whether he is Indian or *gora* (white)—after all he is a man. (Sikh woman, first pregnancy, aged 18).

The Muslim women studied found the internal examination most threatening and in some cases their husbands prevented them going to the hospital for their check-up.

It is not only in the hospital environment that pregnant women feel frightened and bewildered, for throughout the duration of their pregnancy the women have doubts and uncertainties about the birth and their new role as mother. Fears of this kind are often expressed in times of status transformation.

Transition from Pregnancy to Childbirth

This section is concerned with the difference between "becoming" pregnant and "being", or learning how to be a mother. There is also another distinction to be drawn, and that is the comparison between first-time pregnant women for whom the process is a new experience and those women who have been pregnant before. This latter group, although having experienced pregnancy before, may find that this time it is different from the previous one(s) and they may have to change their behaviour accordingly.

Change has a disturbing influence both on the individual and upon social relations. To compensate for these disruptive effects the processes of change are often ritualized, thus giving meaning to unavoidable danger. It is here that Van Gennep's analysis is important because it is related to the dynamic nature of society. It is a dramatic time in the life of the individual and therefore a favourable time for intense education into new roles. For example, the whole purpose of mothercraft classes in Britain is to instruct women how to become "good" mothers. A certain behaviour is expected of the mother-to-be, and for the young woman her first pregnancy denotes the end of childhood.

When I had me first baby I went to the fair and I was you know [pregnant] and things like that—I did go dancing. And me Mum wouldn't believe in it and she said that's why people do have miscarriages. (British working-class woman, first pregnancy, aged 14).

Those without mothers or friends to give positive meaning to pregnancy and birth find them stressful events. The first-time pregnant British women who had been in paid employment before becoming pregnant remarked that on leaving work they experienced social isolation for the first time in their life. This was one aspect of the status transformation they had not anticipated.

> No one explained depression in pregnancy. I'm a very impatient person and it seems such a long time. . . . This is one of the problems, if I'd got more to do—and all my friends, my work friends and that, I've got so far to go . . . and there's none of my old friends around here. . . . I mention it to the family at times, but I haven't told the doctor because there's nothing really you can do about it. (British woman, first pregnancy).

Traditions give meaning to status changes and make the transition easier. Traditions prohibiting certain foods, and actions such as bending, stretching or lifting heavy objects were common to both Asian and British women in the sample. Twenty-four (62%) of the Asian women and 23 (59%) of the British women said they would not lift heavy weights nor do strenuous work. Most often the mother or mother-in-law enforced these prohibitions.

> She [mother] did say not to lift heavy things, or not to overdo it, things like that—or do anything out of the ordinary. Don't do any heavy washing or anything like that. . . . She always used to say, "Take things easy, otherwise you don't know what might happen". (British working-class woman, fourth pregnancy).

> They [mother and mother-in-law] just told me not to pick up weights—lift weights or heavy things. (Sikh woman, second pregnancy).

Some Asian women believed that miscarriage happens when "a barren woman's shadow falls on the pregnant woman", thus reinforcing beliefs about the anti-social powers of childless women. Although nearly all the women studied took precautions to avoid miscarriage, three of the British middle-class women said they would rather miscarry than give birth to a "deformed" child.

> I just felt I knew it all along. I'd got the feeling it wasn't right—some strange reason. I'd got the feeling all the time I was going to lose it for some reason and I was going to start to bleed. I don't know why, I just had you know. (British middle-class woman, previous miscarriage).

> When I did start to miscarry I didn't want to save it. My friend had been in a similar state to me, though slightly later in pregnancy, 'cos I was only nine weeks. And she had taken the advice of her doctor and gone to bed with her feet up for a few days. But I was so frightened that it might be deformed that I wanted it all to come away. (British middle-class woman, previous miscarriage).

Only the British middle-class women articulated preferring to miscarry than give birth to such a child.

Food restrictions were most applicable to the Asian women whose Unani or Ayurvedic system of medicine distinguishes between the heating and cooling effects of foods (see Appendix II and McGilvray, Chapter 2). It is the "hot" foods that are to be avoided during pregnancy, especially during the early months. It is again the mother or mother-in-law who prescribes the food to be eaten.

My mother said not to have "hot" things, not to sit in front of the heater and not to have Coca Cola. . . . The body acquires too much heat and can lead to miscarriage. . . . [Why not the Coca Cola?] Because of the gas in it, in the beginning when the baby is not very secure it can cause miscarriage. (Hindu woman, first pregnancy).

Mother-in-law says "Don't eat too many "hot" things". Things like *sundh* (ginger), garlic and chillies. (Sikh woman, first pregnancy).

Dietary restrictions which the British women observed tended to relate more to those foods thought to cause indigestion and heartburn (e.g. cheese sauce, fried foods). The Asian women also mentioned avoiding these foods. Three British women said they had not eaten "blighted" potatoes as they had heard they could cause spina bifida. Other British women considered that the consumption of alcohol, smoking of cigarettes, the taking of unprescribed drugs and "violent sex" could harm the baby. None of the Asian women smoked and alcohol was rarely consumed.

I haven't taken anything. I haven't even taken an aspirin for a headache, just in case, perhaps its going too far—I don't know. (British women, second pregnancy).

First when I went to the doctor . . . he said about sex. He says you know that sex does not give you a miscarriage, but violent sex does. . . . I was quite surprised because the doctors say, "Oh sex doesn't hurt you". But he was a firm believer that sex could just at the early stages. (British woman, first pregnancy).

The media and members of the medical profession were likely to provide guidelines for the behaviour of British women. For example, in the last quotation the doctor is informing the woman of what is appropriate sexual behaviour for pregnant women, he is also making assumptions about the amount of control the British woman has in determining her sexual relations. Moreover, the British woman who smoked said that pressure to give up was most often exerted by their husbands, or male partner. The man was concerned that the pregnant woman's behaviour may be affecting the future health of *his* child.

Thoughts of the well-being of the unborn child occupy the minds of all expectant mothers at some stage. Some will manipulate their stomach externally to stimulate action if they have not felt the baby move for some time. Others are particularly careful at specific times of the month to ensure that their pregnancy is carried to term. Questions may be asked about the possible deformity of the child, depending on the age and parity of the mother. For instance, among British women third pregnancies are considered to be unlucky.

> If there's going to be something the matter with one of them, like mongolism, it's supposed to come out in the third child. (British woman, third pregnancy).

And some British and Asian women think that their thoughts and feelings can be transported onto the child *in utero.*

> They say that if you see the face of a good thing in the morning you will have a good-looking child. (Sikh woman, third pregnancy).

> If you're happy and relaxed in pregnancy, then the baby will be contented. (British woman, first pregnancy carried to term).

Another area of apprehension relates to the sex of the child and rituals may be performed to determine the sex of the unborn child. This is more likely to be the case where there is a strong preference for a boy or girl, on religious or cultural grounds. In societies such as India, where there is a particular preference for male children, for economic and religious reasons, the woman's status is further enhanced if she bears a son. Twice as many Asian women as British said they would prefer a boy (see Table III).

These figures should be looked at in the context of the sex of the women's existing children. Both groups of multiparous Asian and British women had a total of fifteen boys; whereas the multiparous Asian women had a total of twenty-five girls compared with the British women who had a total of nine. The figures probably reflect the multiparous British women's greater desire for daughters because they were more likely to already have a son and vice versa for the Asian women, although the strong social pressure on Asian women to produce sons should not be forgotten. One first time pregnant Asian woman said:

> He [husband] wants a boy and I want a girl. I prefer a girl. . . . He said, "If it's a boy I'll celebrate, if it's a girl, I won't!" I said, never mind, I'll celebrate. (Hindu woman, first pregnancy).

TABLE III
Respondents' Desired Sex of Child

	Asian		British		Total	
	No.	%	No.	%	No.	%
(a) Final sample						
Male	16	61	8	31	24	46
Female	1	4	15	58	16	31
Do not mind	9	35	3	11	12	23
TOTAL	26	100	26	100	52	100
(b) First-time pregnant women only—final sample						
Desired sex of child						
Male	5	56	2	22	7	39
Female			4	44	4	22
Do not mind	4	44	3	33	7	39
TOTAL	9	100	9	99	18	100

The Asian women who said they did not mind what sex their first child was, made comments such as the following:

Anything will do it's the first one. (Sikh woman, first pregnancy).

It doesn't matter as it's the first one, but I want one of each. (Hindu woman, first pregnancy).

In the Hindu religion it is believed that the time of conception plays a part in determining the sex of the child (Mamdani, 1972). As one young Hindu woman in the study said:

Me mum says if it's moonlight [when conception takes place] it's going to be a boy, and if it's later when it's getting dark then you're going to have a girl. (Hindu woman, first pregnancy).

However, women in the British sample also performed certain rituals to inform them of the sex of the unborn child.

Oh yes, the ring test, my mother-in-law told me about it. She told me about putting your wedding ring (which I can't wear at the moment) on a chain or piece of string, and if it turns to the left it's a boy and if it turns to the right it's a girl. I did it with the first child and it worked. (British middle-class woman, second pregnancy).

Amongst both samples older women had told the pregnant woman what sex of child to expect. The mother-in-law of a Punjabi woman claimed:

I can tell by the face whether a certain lady is going to have a girl or a boy. When the person appears happy she is bound to have a boy, but if she is irritable and grumbles, she will have a girl.

And more universal is the belief amongst Asian women that if the baby is lying on the right side it is a boy and on the left side a girl. This belief is similar to that held by British women when they say that if you carry the baby at the front it will be a boy, and if you carry it all around then it will be a girl.

They [older women] say that if it's on the right side it's a boy, and on the left side a girl—but I can never tell which side the baby is on. (Sikh woman, third pregnancy).

They [older women] say that if your lump's all at the front it's a boy and if it's spread all round it's a girl. (British woman, first pregnancy).

Other beliefs held by the British women refer to the movement of the baby *in utero*; these beliefs strongly reinforce ideas about men being active and women being passive.

> Well I happened to mention it to me mother-in-law when she 'phoned up one day, that . . . er . . . it [the baby] was moving about more. She said it must be a boy. They say boys are more active. (British working-class woman, fourth pregnancy).

> I mean he kicked me so hard he bruised all my stomach and that's another reason why I was convinced when I went into labour that it was a boy. (British working-class woman, fifth pregnancy).

Similarly, the Punjabi women mentioned eating foods that boys like if they are carrying a boy, or even dreaming of such foods.

> Some say that if you are going to have a boy then you feel like having things that boys like. . . . Take, for example, vegetables and lentils and *karhi* [a dish made from gram flour and yoghurt]—if you are going to have a girl then you feel like having these things. Boys like mangoes and pomegranates [symbol of fertility]. Even in the dreams you can see these things. . . . (Sikh woman, fifth pregnancy, four daughters).

Despite all these beliefs surrounding the sex of the child, the pregnant woman's over-riding concern is that the baby will be all right.

> One always keeps wishing to have a boy, but whatever God gives is welcome. (Sikh woman, fifth pregnancy)

> If you have a healthy baby, it doesn't really matter what sex it is. (British woman, third pregnancy).

These comments again reflect different attitudes towards children. The Asian woman was pleased to have any child, but had a definite preference for a boy, the British woman's main concern was that the baby was healthy. However both groups of women knew of things they should avoid if they wanted to prevent giving birth to a handicapped child. The Asian women said they would move around during the *grahan* (an eclipse) and not look at it, while for the British women, exposure to X-rays and eating "diseased" potatoes were seen as particularly harmful.

> They [older women] say that if you look at an eclipse, then the child loses the power of one of his limbs or organs (Sikh woman, fifth pregnancy).

It turned out that I'd been exposed to X-ray right in the very first few weeks of pregnancy. And I was panic striken. . . . I didn't know I was pregnant when I was first X-rayed. I hadn't missed a period then, so that was right at the very dangerous part of pregnancy. This is what worried us. But we were assured that everything would be all right—so I hope he [consultant obstetrician] is right because it's not fair on me or the child if he is wrong. (British working-class woman, fifth pregnancy).

There is a difference between the two groups of women in terms of the amount of retribution they expect when they transgress ritual practices. The Punjabi woman who looks at the *grahan* can expect to give birth to a deformed child, it is in her fate. However, the British woman who is exposed to X-rays early in pregnancy expects members of the medical profession to detect abnormality and to offer her an abortion should any abnormality be diagnosed. In the last instance, it is the doctor who decides whether certain tests should or should not be carried out. If he (all the clinic consultants were male) decides against screening procedures such as amniocentesis, then the woman may continue to worry throughout the pregnancy that something is "wrong" with the baby. This is what happened to the British woman quoted above.

Other British women who were worried about the possibility of the baby being handicapped said they did not receive any reassurance from the hospital antenatal clinic and their husbands were particularly loathe to talk about the subject.

I hope it's all right, that's the thing that worries me. . . . It worries me it really does. I've never spoken about it. If I say to my husband he'll say, "Oh don't be so stupid, why should you?" And it's not a thing you like really to talk about. You're the first person I've really spoken to about that now. . . . (British middle-class woman, third pregnancy).

I think your first thought is, "Well as long as it's all right and everything's there that should be there you know". That's what I've said to me husband many a time and he's said, "Don't talk like that." But I said, "Well you have to face these things." (British working-class woman, first pregnancy).

These comments reinforce the strength of the belief that pregnant women should only think "good" thoughts. To think about a deformity and handicapped children is to tempt fate.

Fatalistic beliefs are most common amongst those people who do not have control over their day-to-day existence. Many of the women, both Asian and British, expressed beliefs about the inevitability of the outcome of their pregnancy. Comments were most often made about the pointlessness of doctors trying to "turn" a breech presentation baby for "it'll only turn back again" or "it will right itself when the time comes". The women persistently argued against induction of labour as "it'll come when it's ready".

The fatalistic beliefs held by Asian women towards miscarriage and stillbirth are most often expressed as "It's God's will", and can best be understood in terms of the high death rates in rural India. Death is a common occurrence over which God has control. The maternal mortality rate in rural India is 23 times as high as the U.K. rate (Morpeth, 1979—figures based on the 1968 census returns). Infant mortality in rural India is six times the rate in the United States, while death in the second year of life in rural India is 27 times greater than in the U.S. (Gordon *et al.*, 1963). However, this belief in the destiny of God does not exclude extensive measures being taken to ward evil away from the expectant woman.

The higher standards of nutrition and housing in industrial societies combined with medical intervention in pregnancy and childbirth have been associated with a decrease in the maternal and perinatal mortality rates.[10] Women in Britain therefore have come to depend on medical intervention in pregnancy and childbirth, often equating hospital confinements with the reduced mortality rates. The Asian women in particular considered hospital deliveries to be safer than home confinements.

Although the mortality rates have decreased there has not been a concomitant increase in preparing women for a medicalized pregnancy and childbirth. First-time pregnant women had very little idea of what it would be like to go into labour:

> Because it's my first chance I don't know anything. (Sikh woman, first pregnancy).

> "No-one's described what the pain should be like." (British woman, first pregnancy).

while those who have given birth before say,

> The question is that the baby should be born with the greatest possible ease, but the babies are always born with pain and trouble. (Muslim woman, sixth pregnancy).

> This time I've had funny fears. The main fear is that it was so painful and so long last time, that even though I'm reassured all round that it won't be so painful, I'm still worried. (British woman, second pregnancy).

The concerns women have about going into labour, coupled with the anxieties about the healthiness of the forthcoming child, are rarely dealt with sensitively in the hospital antenatal clinic setting. In the past these fears were most often allayed by older women who had given birth themselves. The medicalization process undermines the skills of older women and emphasizes the importance of consulting a person who is medically qualified. A contradiction thus arises here between the medical definition of pregnancy as a potentially pathological condition requiring careful and persistent monitoring, and the fact that most of the symptoms presented in pregnancy are considered "normal" to the pregnant state. So when women consult members of the medical profession about their uncertainties they are often consoled with, "There's nothing to worry about". Rarely are they given an explanation for the cause of their concern. This contradiction is again highlighted by the amazing regularity with which pregnant women keep their antenatal appointments. They admit they gain little from these attendances, often involving long waits and abrupt, humiliating examinations. Yet they continue to attend the clinic, because it in some way reassures them, even if it is a negative reassurance: "They would tell me if there was something wrong". Sometimes though, the woman isn't satisfied with this negative reassurance and leaves the clinic distressed, and occasionally in tears.

> Well actually after last week when they upset me at the hospital, I came home and went up to my own doctor that night. I made an appointment because I wanted to know if anything was dreadfully wrong and what they were doing about it. (British woman, third pregnancy—previous stillbirth).

This example shows that the impersonal nature of the hospital clinic does not provide the support and reassurance that most women need. Also it cannot be assumed that these women are receiving support from kin in the social network in modern secular society (Hart, 1976). These observations apply particularly to those Punjabi women in Britain who do not have the support of the extended family and to unmarried British women. However, it is wrong to assume that Punjabi women living in a nuclear family totally lack support. The evidence from this study suggests that these women tend to have a more sharing relationship with their husband (Homans, 1980, pp. 520–522, 531) and the unmarried British women tended to have very close relationships with their mothers.

The professional and lay advice women in Britain receive often depends on their social class, their ethnic background and their linguistic abilities. In this hospital antenatal clinic the absence of an interpreter meant that for the twenty (78%) Asian women who did not speak English fluently, communication was extremely difficult. However, both working-class and middle-class British women experienced difficulty in understanding the doctors at the antenatal clinic.

> I couldn't make out what he was talking about. I had to keep saying "Pardon" and you know, asking him to repeat things and I wasn't really all that clear what he said. (British middle-class woman, third pregnancy).

> Don't ask me about the one I saw on Tuesday because I couldn't understand a word he said. (British working-class woman, fourth pregnancy).

Given the communication problems facing women of different social class and ethnic backgrounds it is not difficult to realize why the women felt constrained in asking for advice or reassurance about any worries they had.

Furthermore, the women's worries were not likely to be allayed at the formal preparation for motherhood classes. I observed these classes over a period of time and analysed their content. The sessions were divided into two parts, one for formal instruction and the other consisted of relaxation exercises to prepare the woman for the birth. The main emphasis in the instruction part of the class was on what to eat during pregnancy; how conception and birth occur; how to feed the baby; how to bath it; what it should wear and how to fold a nappy. The classes were therefore directed at mothercraft, rather than enabling the women to understand the transition in itself. At the end of each class there was time for the women to ask questions and invariably they asked about medical intervention at the time of birth. The particular areas the women expressed interest in were episiotomy, induction of labour, forceps and Caesarian deliveries. However, their questions were rarely answered fully, the midwife in charge nearly always commented that such interventions were unlikely and only happened in extreme cases—apart from episiotomies which are almost routinely carried out "to prevent a nasty tear". However, the national figures for Caesarian section and forceps delivery in 1973 were 5% and 12% respectively (DHSS, 1976) and the local figure for induction in 1976 was 35% of all hospital births. A considerable proportion of women could therefore expect medical intervention in labour and were inadequately prepared for it (see also Hoover-Anwar, 1972; Bacon, 1973/1974; Baric and MacArthur, 1977; Graham, 1976).

Separation of Parturient Women from Society

Throughout the world parturient women are usually separated from ordinary social activities. In rural Punjab the pregnant woman tends to continue her normal duties until the onset of labour. There is a belief that "labour helps labour". Once labour begins, the woman is isolated from the rest of village life. She is within the home, attended by other women, including female relatives and the indigenous midwife (*dai*). The transition to motherhood, while painful, is accomplished in familiar places with familiar people, with a minimum of dislocation. By way of contrast, in industrial societies the woman in hospital is away from her familiar social and domestic environment, subjected to rituals which give her little aid in the social transition to motherhood.

Childbirth is defined in many societies as dangerous, powerful or polluting (Faithorn, 1975, p. 130; Kitzinger, 1978, pp. 226–227; Okely, 1977, p. 68; Chandrasekhar, 1959). It is a time when the woman is not yet a mother, but no longer purely pre-parus. Not fitting clearly within cognitive and social categories, she is in a liminal state, separate from the "safe" categories of ordinary existence. In rites of passage, people at this stage are usually physically separated from ordinary society, as indeed are most women in childbirth (Van Gennep, 1960; Leach, 1976; Douglas, 1966). These attitudes of liminality and marginality are often extended to menstruation, a metaphor for birth. The Sikh religion, for example, does not allow menstruating women to touch the *Guru Granth Sahib* (Holy Book) or attend the Gurdwara (Sikh Temple).

> Then [while menstruating] we can't touch the *Guru Granth Sahib* [Holy Book], my *būa* [father's sister-in-law] told me and also in India I learnt. You can say the words *path* [the Holy words], but you can't touch the book. When they're over [the period] you have a bath and then you can do it [touch the Book]. (Sikh woman, second pregnancy).

The restriction on attending the *Gurdwara* means that Sikh women who are permitted to be priestesses are prevented from conducting their religious duties while menstruating. This reproduces patriarchal social relations by excluding women from certain social activities.

Women of the Hindu religion did not use their Temple as a social gathering place as the Sikh women did and were more likely to pray at home in front of their own home-made Temple. Even then, they would only pray after having a bath. The same restrictions on Temple attendance applied to them when they were menstruating.

> When you have your monthlies you can't go in the Temple, not in our religion. After four or five days you can go, but not before then. You have to have a bath. (Hindu woman, first pregnancy).

The Muslim women were less likely to go to the *Masjid* (mosque).

Only the men go, very few women go. Sometimes we go, but not many women go. (Muslim woman, fourth pregnancy).

Also, like the Hindu women they tended to pray at home, and again they were not able to do this when they were menstruating.

When we have periods, we can't read the Quran [Koran]—but we can read it when we are unwell or pregnant. (Muslim woman, fourth pregnancy).

The Muslim women said there are traditional taboos against menstruating women touching food, cooking and washing clothes. However, none of the Muslim women observed these taboos in Britain. They all lived in nuclear households where they were the only woman attending to the domestic chores.

Although the Asian women said there were no restrictions on them attending their Temple when they were pregnant, when the women were interviewed at eight months pregnant none of the women said they had been to the Temple in the last week. However this was for purely pragmatic reasons as the women have to sit on the floor for the duration of the service.

We try to go every Sunday to the *Gurdwara*—but now I don't go in this condition because I can't sit for long and I find difficulty in getting up. (Sikh woman, fifth pregnancy).

The British women were not aware of religious taboos during menstruation, but they had heard about prohibitions on washing hair and having hot baths. Examples of pollution control in Britain would therefore be the rituals observed when a pregnant woman is admitted to hospital in labour. These include the purging of the body through enemas and catheterization, the cleansing of the body by bathing and the shaving of pubic hairs.

A friend of mine gets her husband to shave her before she goes in. The way they do it, it's embarrassing. You lose your sense of identity. (British working-class woman, fifth pregnancy).

Lomas attributes the passivity of maternity patients in hospital to a female "masochistic urge" which he claims makes them accept "unbiological" behaviour such as the preference for delivery under anaesthesia, separation from their newly delivered baby and the adoption of bottle feeding. However, the passive behaviour of women at this crucial time in their life should not be reduced to a simplistic Freudian analysis which claims that women enjoy suffering and pain. Women do expect childbirth to be painful, but this does not mean that they revel in pain. As an alternative analysis, women's passivity in birth might be viewed in the context of the management of birth. In industrial society, women's inadequate preparation for the transition to motherhood reinforces their passivity in the hospital setting. Their initiation into the role of mother is made more traumatic by the woman's isolation and separation in the labour ward.[11]

> I'd like my husband there. You're left on your own so you might as well have your husband there. But apart from that it could possibly be that they think more of the child if they see it born. I think they're closer to it because they actually see it being born, you know, it's such a marvellous experience. (British woman, first pregnancy).

Five (19%) Asian women and 12 (46%) British women expected their partner to be with them for the birth. The other women said their husband, or male partner, considered childbirth to be women's business, a time of pain and suffering and something which is polluting.

> Who on earth wants to be there? (Traditional Punjabi Muslim woman, fifth pregnancy).

> I think they have funny ideas, I think that they think that there's going to be a lot of blood and mess. (British middle-class woman, third pregnancy).

On the other hand, some women would like to be alone in childbirth, regarding it themselves as a time of impurity.

> I like him [husband] to be there while I'm all nice and decent, but I wouldn't want him there after. (British middle-class woman, fourth pregnancy).

Reluctance on the part of husbands to attend the birth is most marked amongst "traditional" Asian men, and their wives will say, "He doesn't want to stay himself". "Traditional" in this context refers to those Asians with little or no command of the English language who live in an extended family. They tend to follow the rules that would apply in rural India, where birth is women's business and all men are excluded. However, less traditional Asian women, that is those educated in this country and living in a nuclear family, are more likely to want their husbands with them at birth, for comfort and support.

> I don't mind my mother or him [husband], but I would like someone there to encourage me. (First time pregnant English-speaking Hindu woman, living in a nuclear family).

Also non-English speaking Asian women would often like someone with them in labour to translate for them. Those British women who have seen films of the birth of a baby and not been deterred by them, and who also have a sharing relationship with their husband are likely to want him to participate in the event.

> I think it does them good to see it personally. Well it makes you both closer because you're going through it all together, as a family. . . . I'd like him to be there seeing the birth, even a Caesarian. I don't know why they don't let them watch actually, as long as they're sterile and what have you, which they have to be anyway when they go in to watch you having a baby. . . . (First time pregnant British woman).

The above examples depict how pregnant women from two different ethnic backgrounds, but now residing in the same country, react to the separation of childbirth from the rest of society. The differences and similarities between the two groups of women are significant. The more traditional women from both samples seem to accept that childbirth in Britain should be set apart from home, family and friends, whilst the less traditional women are wanting to share their birth experience with others from their personal social circle.

Re-integration of the Mother into Society

Van Gennep recognized the social as well as the physical components of childbirth.

> It is apparent that the physiological return from childbirth is not the primary consideration, but that instead there is a *social return* from childbirth, just as there is a social parenthood which is distinct from sexual union (Van Gennep, 1960, p. 46).

The social return of the women from childbirth, the final ceremony in the "rite of passage" seems to have lost some of its significance in Britain today. The ceremony of the re-integration of the woman back into her family now occurs at the entrance to the hospital where the maternity sister hands over the baby to the mother (or sometimes to the father) before they leave. The ceremony that used to be significant at this time was the "churching of women" in which the woman gives her thanks to God for delivering her from the "great pain and peril of childbirth" (Book of Common Prayer). It also marks the end of her period of potential pollution and is the final cleansing act before her re-integration into society. Although this ceremony has lost most of its significance, women who are in hospital the Sunday following birth are often invited to give thanks to God in the hospital chapel. Other religious women may go to their own church soon after discharge, though the numbers are likely to be few. (Of the sample only three (11%) British women interviewed said that they intended to be "churched" or attend chapel or church soon after delivery.)

> Me mum wants me to be churched, she's already mentioned it. I'll do it just to shut her up. (Young unmarried British woman).

Another woman said she had received a prayer asking for her safe delivery through childbirth.

> During my first pregnancy my mother-in-law sent me a little card which I found upstairs a few weeks ago. . . . It was to Saint Anthony, a prayer that I might be spared the pains and agonies of childbirth, which I thought was the most tactless thing to send. (British middle-class woman, second pregnancy).

The re-integration into society of the newly delivered woman in rural India is marked more clearly by rituals which are related to the period of impurity. The woman's period of impurity varies from ten days among the Brahmins to 40 days among the lower castes. Traditionally neither the woman nor the child should come out of the confinement room during this period (Chandrasekhar, 1959). For women of all castes the total period of confinement lasts for 40 days after which the woman can resume her normal duties. The extent to which Punjabi women in Britain observe the 40 day period of confinement depends on the presence of other women in the household, particularly the mother-in-law, and the economic situation of the household.

> Mother-in-law, she won't let me out of this house for 40 days anyway. Last time I went to bed for 40 days. . . . After 40 days go to the Temple and take blessing from there—then you can go anywhere. Bless baby as well and baby's name chosen from the Holy Book. (Young English speaking Punjabi Hindu woman, second pregnancy, living in extended family).

> My mother-in-law tried her best to give me complete rest for six weeks, but I didn't want to give her too much burden with the housework. After the first delivery I did take six weeks rest, but after having other children I try to help my mother-in-law in looking after the children. But in the housework, she did not let me help her. (Punjabi Sikh woman, fourth pregnancy, living in extended family).

Asian women who do not live in extended families (58% of the sample studied) find it difficult to arrange for help after they come out of hospital.

It is difficult because there is no mother-in-law here [in Britain]. It is difficult for my mother to come because she has to look after her grandsons—her daughter-in-law goes to work. My brothers are small too and father goes to work, so it is difficult for her. My mother wants me to go to her so that she can look after me, but I'm all right here, I don't want to go there. (Punjabi Sikh woman, sixth pregnancy, living in nuclear family).

The absence of kin in this country was one of the reasons the Asian women cited when they said they would prefer a hospital delivery. The other reasons were that they thought the hospital was "safer" and hospital services in Britain are free. Only one Asian and one British woman said they wanted a home delivery.[12]

Apparently Asian traditional rituals surrounding re-integration of the newly delivered woman into society are breaking down in Britain. However, amongst the British middle-class women new rituals seem to be developing. For instance, these women mentioned their own anxiety about how existing children would respond to the new arrival. They were therefore more concerned about the integration of the new baby into the original family.

Well she's only 21 months [daughter], she knows, well she keeps saying there's a baby in here [points to bulge], but um . . . how much she understands I don't know. I've tried to let her see as many small babies as possible. She knows the baby's room, but how much she understands about it I don't know. I'm a bit apprehensive about how she's going to react, it's difficult. (British middle-class woman, second pregnancy).

Another woman described an even more detailed ritual she had planned to aid the new baby's integration and avoid sibling jealousy.

At the moment I'm in the process of getting her [daughter] a little doll with a bath and its own dummy, so that she can copy. She always wants to help. . . . What I want to do with the doll and what have you, is to take it into hospital with me so that when she comes to visit me the first time to see the baby, I'm going to give it to her and say, "Well this is your baby of your own and you can help me with this one at home." And hopefully we can stop any feelings of jealousy. (British middle-class woman, second pregnancy).

The working-class women on the other hand, were more pragmatic about the integration of the new-born into the family. This can perhaps be related to the larger family size and lack of funds to provide baby-substitutes. However, they did mention devising their own rituals.

What I normally do to get over it [the fact that children are not allowed to touch the baby in the hospital]—when I get home I line them up, put them on the settee and as soon as I get home I give them the baby. Make them feel that it is their baby. I mean it is their baby, they've got to learn to live with it. (British working-class woman, fifth pregnancy).

I would argue that the re-integration of the newly delivered woman, and the integration of the newborn baby, into the home and family need to be treated more sensitively than at present. For example, those women who have had "unsuccessful" pregnancies, i.e. a miscarriage or a stillbirth, do not receive sufficient support or counselling which would help to allay some of their fears and aid their re-integration. Lewis (1976) highlights the doctor's reluctance to console the woman who has had a stillbirth. He says there is a strong pressure on professionals "to keep the crisis of stillbirth hidden away, thereby in fact hindering the mourning and healing process" (1976, pp. 619–620; Jones, Chapter 10).

Moreover women who experience a successful outcome to their pregnancy are still insufficiently prepared for motherhood. They may suffer from puerperal depression, and those who want to breastfeed may experience difficulty and discomfort in doing so. This is particularly significant in British society where many women work outside of the home until the birth of their first child, after the birth they feel isolated and may experience a "loss of self identity". For instance, Oakley (1980, p. 213) refers to the "bereavement" newly delivered women experience.

Conclusion

This chapter has argued that an analysis of pregnancy and birth as a rite of passage is only useful if it incorporates into the analysis the viewpoint of the women concerned. To become a mother has different meanings to women in industrial society, depending on their social class and ethnic background.

All the women studied observed some rituals during their passage to motherhood. The Asian women living in extended families were more likely to be compelled to observe these rituals by their mother-in-law. However, some of the British women devised their own rituals as a means of coping with the period of uncertainty. The rituals to do with determining the sex of the child *in utero* are remarkably similar for all the women studied. Those rituals to do with religion and food are more obviously culturally prescribed. Moreover, the common assumptions that "old wives' tales" and superstitions are only taken seriously by the uneducated or uninformed is called into question. Of the British sample, highly educated women, those who had been to college or university, were as likely to express knowledge of and some belief in, the rituals surrounding pregnancy as were the less educated women. The same was true for educated Asian women. However, the more educated women were also likely to be familiar with medical knowledge and to be more critical of the treatment they received. The less educated women were more likely to be dependent on members of the medical profession as they did not have the knowledge to question advice given. Furthermore, it would appear that as all pregnant women of whatever social class and ethnic background observe some rituals during pregnancy, face uncertainty and have both specific and nameless fears, there is therefore a need for the medical profession in Britain to address itself to these areas rather than an exclusive focus on the clinical or pathological condition.

The transition through pregnancy to motherhood and its attendant uncertainities must be treated sensitively if there is any concern for the emotional well-being of the mother. The medical profession has assumed command of childbirth without recognizing that it is also a social event. At present the care that a woman receives during the antenatal period varies considerably with her culture, class and linguistic ability. For instance, the most prestigious fee-paying antenatal classes run by the National Childbirth Trust were attended by a few white middle-class women. The non fee-paying local authority run classes were attended by nearly all the first-time pregnant British women but only two English-speaking Asian women. They were the only Asian women who had any formal preparation for childbirth and motherhood. The inappropriateness of antenatal care for the vast majority of Asian women reinforces an overdependence upon the doctor. As one Asian woman said:

> It is true that the doctor is everything for the patient when she is in pain . . . the woman is in such a condition that the doctor becomes everything for her.

Acknowledgements

An earlier version of this chapter was first presented to the British Medical Anthropology Society Meeting on Childbirth in January 1978. It forms part of my Ph.D. thesis supervised by Professor Margaret Stacey, and funded by the S.S.R.C. The use of an interpreter was made possible by a grant from the Health Education Council. I would like to thank especially Margaret Stacey, Carol MacCormack and Hilary Graham for their comments on an earlier draft of the paper, Bhupinder Dhesi for her interpreting services and insight into Asian culture, the Birmingham Interpreting and Translating Service for their translating and transcribing. Finally, thanks to all the women involved in the study.

Notes

(1) Gluckman (1966) develops these ideas further in "Essays of the Ritual of Social Relations": Manchester University Press.

(2) Hereafter referred to as Asian. Although the distinction is made in this paper between Asian and British women, this is not to deny Asian women their British citizenship. The dichotomy is cultural, made for descriptive and comparative purposes.

(3) In the city studied 80% of all known antenatal patients received their antenatal care from both their general practitioner (G.P.) and the hospital consultant clinic. This system of antenatal care is commonly known as "shared" care. The women who receive this kind of care give birth in the consultant wards of the maternity hospital. All the women studied in this research fall into this category. The other known antenatal patients (20%) were those who had been screened and deemed to be less "at risk" and not requiring specialist care. They received all their antenatal care from their G.P. and gave birth in the G.P. unit of the maternity hospital. At the time of the study less than 1% of births were home deliveries where the woman gave birth at home with a domiciliary midwife (and sometimes the G.P.) in attendance. Home births have decreased tremendously since the building of a new maternity hospital in 1966. At that time there were 50% home confinements and the number has fallen to less than 1% by 1976. About 6% of women per year gave birth in hospital without receiving any antenatal care at all.

(4) Two of the Asian women had migrated to Britian when they were pregnant—one at four months pregnant and the other one at seven and a half months pregnant.

(5) Although about 40% of British women work outside the home they tend to be poorly paid, in service rather than production jobs, and seldom have managerial status.

(6) Of the 19 Punjabi women, 11 came from the *Jat* caste; two came from the *Chohra* (untouchable) caste; one from the *Ramgharia* (skilled artisans, e.g. carpenter) caste; two from agricultural labourer caste

(i.e. working for Jats); two Hindu women from the small business/ shopkeeping caste and one Hindu woman was a Brahmin.

The other seven women were either Gujerati Hindus of small business/shopkeeping (caste)—two women; one educated Muslim woman; one Muslim woman from agricultural labourer family and three Hindu women who had come to Britian via East Africa—one came from a business family in Uganda and the other two were from agricultural families.

(7) For a discussion of home-workers in North London see Hope *et al.* (1976). Barker and Allen (also 1976, p. 7) say of the women portrayed in this article, "Many of these women are encapsulated in a contradiction between the good wife and mother ideology and the sheer material necessities of day to day living".

(8) Guillebaud (16 November 1955)—Report of the Committee of Enquiry into the Cost of the N.H.S. 1953–1956. H.M.S.O. Cmd. 9663. This report attempts to rationalize supplies and to make use of existing resources more efficiently through centralization, e.g. impose hospital accounting systems, centralized laundries, large scale canteens. Argues for economies of scale.

Cranbrook (27 November 1958)—Report of the Maternity Services Committee (32-455)—established to examine the British Maternity Services, highlights the problems encountered with having home and hospital deliveries within a tripartite system. Sees the unification of maternity services as an ultimate goal and argues for 70% hospitalization of all births.

Peel (1970)—Domiciliary Midwifery and Maternity Bed Needs (Report of the Sub-Committee)—argues that the Perinatal Mortality Survey demonstrated that women were being booked for delivery at home who might reasonably be expected to experience complications in labour, and as a result were having to be transferred to hospital at a late stage, with enhanced risk to mother and child. It advocates unification of maternity services with 100% hospital confinement.

(9) A possible explanation for the Asian women's lack of criticism of the long waits at the clinic may be related to their knowledge of the hospital services in India where people wait up to a day to be seen and even then may have to go again the following day.

(10) There is considerable controversy over the relationship between medical intervention (and hospitalization of births) and the post-war reduction in perinatal mortality. Cochrane (1972) argues that it is not sufficient to say that because two factors (i.e. hospitalization of births and the perinatal mortality rate) co-vary they are

correlated, without taking into account other factors. Moreover, the hospital as the "correct" place of birth has been seriously questioned by Kitzinger and Davis (1978).

(11) It is only recently that the maternity hospital studied permitted husbands to accompany their wives in labour. Even now it is only husbands who are allowed into the delivery room—mothers, boy-friends and women friends are not allowed. After delivery the visiting hours are such that only husbands can visit in the evening 7-8 p.m. while anyone else can visit between 3 and 4 p.m. Visitors (including husbands and other children) are not permitted to pick up the baby in hospital—the hospital considering this to introduce infection (see Homans, 1980, pp. 537–543).

(12) The possibility of obtaining a home delivery is now very slight and it is only those women who are (1) medically screened as suitable and (2) determined to fight for a home confinement (which may involve changing G.P.) who will obtain one.

References

Bacon, L. (1973/1974). "Early Motherhood, Accelerated Role Transition and Social Pathologies". *Social Forces* **52**, 333–341.

Baric, L. and MacArthur, C. (1977). "Health Norms in Pregnancy". *British Journal of Preventive and Social Medicine* **31**, 30–38.

Beechey, V. (1977). "Some Notes on Female Wage Labour in Capitalist Production". *Capital and Class*, No. 3, Autumn, 45–66.

Beveridge, W. (1942). Social Insurance and Allied Services: The Beveridge Report, Command No. 6404, London: HMSO.

Bowlby, J. (1951). Maternal Health and Mental Health. Geneva: WHO.

Butler, N. R. and Bonham, D. G. (1963). *Perinatal Mortality*. Edinburgh: E. & S. Livingstone.

Carlebach, J. (1966). "Tribal Customs Associated with Pregnancy". *Mother and Child* **36**, 9–13.

Chandrasekhar, S. (1959). *Infant Mortality in India 1901–1955*. London: George Allen & Unwin.

Cochrane, A. L. (1972). *Effectiveness and Efficiency: Random Reflections on Health Services*. London: Oxford University Press.

Common Prayer, Book of, p. 232. London: Eyre & Spottiswoode.

Department of Health and Social Security (1976). On the State of Public Health. Report to the Chief Medical Officer for 1974. London: HMSO.

Douglas, M. (1966). *Purity and Danger*. London: Routledge & Kegan Paul.

Faithorn, E. (1975). "The Concept of Pollution among the Kafe of the Papua New Guinea Highlands". In *Toward an Anthropology of Women* (R. Reiter, ed.). New York: Monthly Review Press.

Ford, C. S. (1964). A Comparative Study of Reproduction. New Haven: Human Relations Area Files Press.

Freedman, L. and Ferguson, V. (1949). "The Question of Painless Childbirth in Primitive Cultures". Yale University Annual Meeting.

Galloway, J. (1965). "Immigration in the Midlands". *Lancet*, 9 October, p. 731.

Galloway, J. (1968). "Domiciliary Midwifery in Wolverhampton". *Lancet*, 26 October, p. 906.

Gideon, H. (1962). "A Baby is Born in the Punjab". *American Anthropologist* **64**, 1220–1234.

Gill, D. G., Illsley, R. and Koplick, L. H. (1970). "Pregnancy in Teenage Girls". *Social Science and Medicine* **3**, 549–574.

Gordon, J. E., Chitkara, I. D. and Wyon, J. B. (1963). "Preventive Medicine and Epidemiology". *The American Journal of the Medical Sciences* **245**, 345–377.

Graham, H. (1976). "The Social Image of Pregnancy: Pregnancy as a Spirit Possession". *Sociological Review* **24**, 291–308.

Hart, N. (1976). *When Marriage Ends: A Study in Status Passage*. London: Tavistock Publications.

Henslin, J. and Biggs, M. A. (eds) (1971). *Studies in the Sociology of Sex*. New York: Appleton–Century–Crofts.

Homans, H. (1980). "Pregnant in Britain: A Sociological Approach to Asian and British Women's Experiences". Unpublished Ph.D. Thesis, University of Warwick.

Hope, E. *et al.* (1976). "Home-workers in North London". In *Dependence and Exploitation in Work and Marriage* (D. Barker and S. Allen, eds). London: Longman.

Hoover-Anwar, R. A. (1972). "Coping with the Crisis of Pregnancy: Explorations of the Interactive Network Among Married and Unmarried Mothers". Ph.D. Thesis, University of London.

Joseph, K. (1974). Speech. 19 October. Birmingham.

Kitzinger, S. (1978). *Women as Mothers*. Glasgow: Fontana.

Kitzinger, S. and Davis, J. A. (1978). *The Place of Birth*. Oxford: Oxford University Press.

Land, H. (1976). "Women: Supporters or Supported?" In *Sexual Divisions and Society: Process and Change* (D. Barker and S. Allen, eds). London: Tavistock Publications.

Leach, E. R. (1976). *Culture and Communication: The Logic by which Symbols are Connected*. Cambridge: Cambridge University Press.

Lewis, E. (1976). "The Management of Stillbirth: Coping with an Unreality". *Lancet*, 18 September, 619–620.

Lewis, O. (1965). *Village Life in Northern India*. New York: Vintage Books.

Lomas, P. (1966). "Ritualistic Elements in the Management of Childbirth". *British Journal of Medical Psychology* **39**, 207–213.

McIntyre, S. (1975). "Decision Making Processes Following Pre-marital Conception". Ph.D. Thesis, Aberdeen.

McIntyre, S. (1977). *Single and Pregnant*. London: Croom Helm.

McKinlay, J. B. (1970). "A Brief Description of a Study on the Utilization of Maternity and Child Welfare Services by the Lower Working Class Sub-Culture". *Social Science and Medicine* **4**, 551–556.

McKinlay, J. B. (1972). "Some Social Characteristics of Lower Working Utilizers and Underutilizers of Maternity Care Services". *Journal of Health and Social Behaviour* **13**, 369–382.

Mamdani, Mahmood (1972). *The Myth of Population Control: Family, Caste and Class in an Indian Village*. New York: Monthly Review Press.

Marshall, J. F. (1973). "Culture and Contraception". D. Phil. Thesis in Anthropology, University of Hawaii.

Milio, N. (1975). "Values, Social Class and Community Health Services". In Sociology of Medical Practice (C. Cox and A. Mead, eds). London: Collier-Macmillan.

Morpeth, R. (1979). "The Village Midwife in the Punjab". Unpublished paper, Cambridge.

Moyes, B. (1977). "A Doctor is a Doctor". New Society, 10 November, pp. 289–291.

Myrdal, A. and Klein, V. (1956). Women's Two Roles. London: Routledge and Kegan Paul.

Newman, L. F. (1969). "Folklore of Pregnancy: Wives Tales in Contra Costa Country, California". Western Folklore, XXVIII, 112–135.

Newton, J. R. (1979). "The Future of Gynaecology". Paper given at Human Relations in Obstetric Practice Seminar, University of Warwick, 19th March.

Oakley, A. (1976). "Wisewoman and Medicine Man". In The Rights and Wrongs of Women (J. Mitchell and A. Oakley, eds). Harmondsworth: Penguin.

Oakley, A. (1980). Women Confined: Towards a Sociology of Childbirth. London: Martin Robertson.

Okeley, J. (1977). "Gypsy Women: Models in Conflict". In Perceiving Women (S. Ardener, ed.). New York: Halstead.

Paige, K. E. and Jeffrey, M. (1973). "The Politics of Birth Practices: A Strategic Analysis". American Sociological Review 38, 663–677.

Pearson, J. F. (1973). "Social and Psychological Aspects of Extra-marital First Conceptions". Journal of Bio-Social Science 5, 453–496.

Peck, E. (1973). The Baby Trap? London: Heinrich Hanau.

Pickering, W. S. F. (1974). "The Persistence of Rites de Passage: Towards an Explanation". British Journal of Sociology 25, 63–78.

Powell, E. (1969). In Freedom and Reality, pp. 307–308. Surrey: Paperfronts, Elliot Right Way Books.

Saunders, L. (1954). Cultural Differences and Medical Care. New York: Russell Sage Foundation.

Smith, A. (1970). "Progress in the 1960s and Problems for the 1970s". In In the Beginning: Studies of Maternity Services (G. McLachlan and R. Shegog, eds). Oxford: Oxford University Press.

Stevens, B. (1971). "Psychoses Associated with Childbirth: A Demographic Survey". Social Science and Medicine 5, 527–543.

Van Gennep, A. V. (1960). The Rites of Passage. Chicago: University of Chicago Press. (English translation). 1st Edition 1908.

Weeks, J. R. (1976). "Infant Mortality and Premarital Pregnancies". Social Science and Medicine 10, 165–169.

Appendix I

Things to be Avoided Whilst Pregnant

Asian Women, *n* = 39*

    Lifting heavy things—mentioned by 22 women ⎤   24

    Doing heavy work—mentioned by 2 women ⎦ women

Straining the body

Running

Sitting during an eclipse—must walk around and not look at it otherwise
    it will affect the baby

Having tight clothing around the waist—may affect the baby

Eating "hot" curries

Eating "hot" stuff—particularly chillies, peppers

Eating "hot" food—may lose the baby

Eating "sour" things

Eating fried foods

British women, *n* = 39*

    Lifting heavy things—mentioned by 15 women ⎤   23

    Anything strenuous—mentioned by 5 women ⎬ women

    Doing heavy work—mentioned by 3 women ⎦

Stretching

Running about

"Overdoing" it

Horse-riding

Netball

Putting on too much weight

Excesses of food and drink

X-rays

Drugs

Smoking

Fried foods

Blighted potatoes

Violent sex

Wearing high-heeled shoes

* Some women advocated "avoiding" more than one thing, whilst a
few women considered that they should "carry on as normal" when
pregnant.

Note: The similarity between the two samples in terms of not lifting
heavy things or doing heavy work.

Appendix II

Classification of Some Food According to the Ayurvedic Tradition

"Hot" foods	*"Cold" foods*
Chilli	Boiled rice
Tumeric	Blackgram
Wheat	Cow milk
Mustard seeds	Buffalo milk
Garlic	Butter milk
Chicken	Ghee
Honey	Banana
Potato	Black pepper
Fish	Tea
Horse gram	Onion
Groundnut	Peas
Drumstick	Oranges
Bitter gourd	Pumpkin
Carrot	Green tomatoes
Radish	Spinach
Fenugreek	Guava
Green mango	Greengram
Paw-paw	
Dates	
Coffee	
Ginger	
Egg	

References

Aman (1969). *Medicinal Secrets of Your Food*. 1st edition, Mysore, India.
Nichter, M. (1977). "Health Ideologies and Medical Cultures in the South Kanara Areca-Nut Belt". Unpublished Ph.D. Thesis, Edinburgh.
Ramanamurthy, P. S. V. (1969). *Journal of Nutrition and Diet* **6**, 187.
Shah, P. M. (1975). *Indian Paediatrics* **12**, 73.

10. Childbirth in a Scientific and Industrial Society*

A. D. JONES

AND

C. DOUGHERTY

This chapter is concerned with childbirth in industrial societies, mainly in Western Europe and North America where the circumstances surrounding childbearing are characterized by a number of features, typically (a) an interest by the medical professions as experts, (b) heterogeneous customs and attitudes among pregnant women reflecting a wide range of desires concerning the management of pregnancy, delivery and postnatal care, (c) choice of preparation, especially in attendance at antenatal classes. The way in which these features facilitate the development of the young adult into parenthood in modern industrial culture is important both for those people themselves and for those who seek to emulate them.

*We would like to thank Professor Norman Morris and the staff and patients at the Department of Obstetrics, the Charing Cross Hospital, West London, for their help and encouragement in the preparation of the material for this chapter. The study was funded by the Social Research Fund of the London School of Economics and Political Science.

259

The Medical Interest

The medical profession has increased its interest in childbirth (Kitzinger and Davis, 1978). In industrialized countries a high proportion of births occur in hospital. In countries with the lowest figure the proportion is about a half and these account for most first births. The first transition to parenthood is very likely, then, to occur in a hospital. Several visits will have been made to doctors during pregnancy and a few days will be spent in a hospital ward postnatally. Obstetricians are encouraged in their efforts to increase their interest in managing childbirth by the knowledge and belief that they were able to reduce perinatal mortality and morbidity in both mother and child and that they are able to reduce painful suffering by the uses of drugs. Chard and Richards (1977) and Kitzinger and Davis (1978) discuss the trends in medical practice and effectiveness. Some of the changes which have occurred in health and well-being can be attributed, in part, to obstetric practice and, in part, to changes in diet, stature, drug addiction (especially nicotine), family size and poverty. Hospitalization and medical intervention carry their own risks, especially to the mental state of the mother-to-be and to the initial condition of the baby if drugs have been used. Although conflict of interest has arisen between different medical professions, notably between obstetricians and midwives (Donnison, 1977), and paediatricians, the tendency has been to bring more aspects of pregnancy under medical supervision. Paramedical personnel have in some cases shared an interest in this. Physiotherapists working in hospitals and clinics established in medical institutions hold meetings at which pregnant women, usually in the third trimester, learn techniques of relaxation and muscular control to reduce pain in labour thus tending to bring under medical auspices procedures having their origin outside the conceptual reference of medicine. Russian (Velvosky, 1972), French (Leboyer, 1975; Lamaze, 1958) and British (Dick-Read, 1933) writers have influenced attempts to help and train women to control their own bodies during labour using psychoprophylactic methods. Other influences appear to have an oriental origin and to have been mediated by experts in the practice of Yoga.

In Britain all women are entitled to free medical care antenatally, during birth and postnatally. Family doctors and hospitals provide antenatal care. Nearly all births occur in hospital and postnatal check-ups are carried out by both hospital and family doctors. Health visitors, who are trained in midwifery, also visit the woman's home. In maternity hospitals the actual birth is supervised by midwives, who in addition to being qualified as nurses, have a training in midwifery and can administer certain drugs without the authorization of a doctor. (Nurses may not do this.) Doctors are only called to a woman in labour if the midwife thinks it necessary or if, due to her medical or obstetric history, the doctor decides he should take an active interest in the birth himself. Hospitals and some private organizations run classes to prepare pregnant women for childbearing. The National Childbirth Trust is by far the largest of these organizations and, unlike the hospitals and family doctors, they charge a fee.

The increase in the medical interest in childbirth places a burden on medical staff during childbirth. This burden concerns both the emotions surrounding failure in childbirth, notably stillbirth and neonatal death, and the paradoxes that the "patients" in their care are not "invalids" or "ill". Menzies (1960) argues that fear of responsibility for patients' suffering and guilt feelings about failure to prevent it lead to actions which defend medical staff against the psychological disturbance of working in an atmosphere highly charged with anxiety. These actions, routinization, secrecy and depersonalization prevent the staff from becoming upset and enable them to continue working at tasks some of which are highly disagreeable. The behaviour of the staff can, however, help or hinder the transition which women make into maternal identity which is discussed later in this chapter.

Although the experience for the "patient" is heightened and of great import, the relationship with the staff is established and completed with the task done or handed over to a colleague in rather less than eight hours which is the usual length of a hospital shift. Under these circumstances recourse to stereotyping, and error in understanding the significance of what a person says or does, is likely to be high even among intelligent and experienced staff who are themselves well adjusted emotionally. The burden which these factors place on staff is severe. If childbirth were not also highly charged with joy at a successful birth, morale among maternity hospital staff would become a serious problem. Staff frequently show signs of ambivalence about their own interventions and experience joy at a birth in which there are none, when the mother "pushes her baby out herself" and when she may be under "stress" but well able to cope without signs of "distress" which are alarming to patients and staff alike.

Stereotyping and misunderstanding something about the situation affects both staff and patients. The following are some examples.

(a) *Skin colour cue.* Doctor and midwife leave the room after a vaginal examination leaving the patient, the ward sister (who is black and originally from Jamaica and with many years of experience as a midwife and several years being responsible for a busy labour ward) and an 18-year-old white student nurse. The sister asked the patient how she felt. "I think I'm doing all right at the moment" was the reply. "But (and this was said turning head and eyes away from the sister to the young student), I am not sure what is happening. How long is this going to last?" The student nurse did not expect to be able to answer this sort of question and by gesture quickly deferred to her senior and qualified colleague. The patient had made the error of assuming that the white nurse was the best source of information. (This error is not at all infrequent.)

(b) *Significance of raised voices.* A patient had asked the midwife on a number of occasions during the first stage of labour to "keep me in the picture and tell me what to do". Everything went very harmoniously until during the second stage the midwife told the patient loudly to push harder and continued to urge her vigorously. Some women, perhaps with a sense of performance and the imminence of a great achievement, like to be shouted on and respond with a lot of effort. On this occasion the woman did not. She wanted to concentrate on pushing without distraction and said, "You keep on doing that. I wish you wouldn't shout so. It is silly. You are taking my mind off it." The words and the tone of voice broke the rapport with the midwife.

These types of interpersonal misunderstanding are fairly common even among well adjusted and experienced women because they do not have the opportunity to get to know one another before they meet in the labour ward. Some problems between staff and patient lie more deeply in the personality of those involved.

Two examples of women unable to relate to anyone helping them during pregnancy and labour illustrate problems which demand a disproportionate effort on the part of the staff. The lives of both these women were characterized by impoverished relationships and unusual demands on other people.

(a) A woman in her thirties whose first marriage ended in separation after six months followed by divorce. She was brought to the U.K. as a fiancée but left the man after a few months living in his flat. She later married a rich businessman. Two attempts to take a degree were each abandoned after a few terms. An attempt to become a physiotherapist was also abandoned. She had been very upset at the death of her own mother. She expected her father to visit her from his home in Spain if she wanted to see him and continued to ask him for money although her second marriage made this unnecessary. She continued her passive support of a left wing group dedicated to the destruction of the present economic and social order.

Her pregnancy was confirmed at about eight weeks and she booked into a hospital. Dissatisfaction led to a change of hospitals and at 30 weeks she booked into another hospital. She attended frequently in order to impress upon the staff that it was essential that her baby was delivered by Caesarean. She showed much charm and warmth during this period and said in a very convincing way that she knew it was irrational but her mother, other relatives and many friends had all suffered so much in labour that she felt she was going to be permanently damaged or die. Her communications with the hospital were frequent; three or more times a week. The consultant, committed normally to as little interference as possible, consented to help her cope with her irrational fears in an otherwise normal and wanted pregnancy by arranging a Caesarean section under general anaesthetic during the forty-first week of pregnancy.

Two days later the patient said she had had a Caesarean to avoid pain in labour and to get her figure back again, but that she was now in greater pain than was right and she complained. She warmly praised the nursing staff about their care for her and her baby and received a great deal of attention in the initial post-delivery period. On the second day, however, she said she could not be expected to ruin her figure by breast feeding and requested treatment to inhibit lactation and reduce her breast size. Suggestions that breast feeding, in addition to being good for the baby, helped restoration of the body were rejected and she became angry at what she thought was unnecessary delay in meeting her request. Subsequently she complained vehemently that the nursing staff were not looking after her or considering her feelings and that they did things to her baby without consulting her. She confronted staff on the ward about these matters ignoring on a number of occasions her own baby who was crying in a way indicative of a typical neonate's need for food, holding and removal of excreta. She developed the habit of perfuming her baby with various powders and scents and discharged herself early with a warm display of gratitude and gifts to the ward staff whom she also chided for taking life too seriously.

(b) A woman in her late twenties who already had two children aged 9 and 7 who lived abroad with her ex-husband and his second wife. A strikingly attractive woman in the style of the 1960s who said she was an actress really but who had not needed to train and who had not yet been discovered. She lived "in a commune", was without any political views and believed that there should be no division between experts and clientele. Doctors should be abolished and birth should be natural in the sense that its management should not be elaborate, technical or rehearsed but should unfold in a biological way. Certain natural aids, mainly herbal, might be tried by those who felt inclined, such as marigold flower oil to anoint the perineum. Attendance for antenatal care was marked by not keeping appointments. Having said she would not attend any antenatal classes she attended irregularly on one or two occasions in each of five separate classes which were running at the hospital at various points during the last ten weeks of her pregnancy. Her presence was often disruptive as, in addition to being an obvious and endlessly apologetic intruder, she interjected remarks which distracted the teacher. "Surely it was you who said last week that some doctors get scissor happy" (referring to episiotomies); "Ooh! I think if a midwife *touched* me when I was giving birth I would kick her, hard, right away so she wouldn't come back." "You are trying to infantilize us all aren't you?"

It became apparent that this woman was unable to get a firm commitment from anyone to accompany her throughout labour as a birth partner. She contacted the National Childbirth Trust to provide one. Throughout most of labour she whimpered and dismissed or ignored attempts to communicate with her and swore at the birth partner provided for her.

Postnatally she was pleased with her baby but she thought it was too greedy and fed too much. Although she liked the idea of supplementing breast feeding with bottle feeds she thought that water was to be discouraged. She liked cradling her baby but avoided changing his nappy. When discharge was discussed she said she could not leave until her accommodation was rearranged as she had been told to leave her present dwelling. Part of her possessions were in a trunk in the "left luggage" at Waterloo Station. She had no definite plans yet where to live but was sure something would turn up. She was not keen to see a social worker but was gentle and frank when one visited her. When she left the hospital, to stay with a friend, she said she was pleased she had had no drugs as a hospital once gave her a "shot of something or other" which had changed her completely so that her life "was all a hallucination".

These types of patient accentuate the tendency of staff to be on their guard against patients who are very difficult to manage. In extreme cases hospital staff can come to view any questioning or assertion of choice by the patient as a sign that she is going to be hostile, uncoop-erative and difficult to help. There is then a tendency to preempt dif-ficulties by gaining maximum control over the woman who is forced into submission.

The Management of Birth

Fertility and birth are features of life where the rational mode of belief is in competition with experience and personal identity. There is an emphasis on scientific method in industrial countries. Ideas are, in principle, put to the test, rigorously studied and modified where the facts dictate. Explanations are given in terms of mechanical relationships between physical entities. Women believe that conception, pregnancy and birth are controlled by body chemistry. Knowledge of body chem-istry is the speciality of doctors after a long training and is increasing due to researchers using scientific methods. The management of birth is the responsibility of obstetric and mid-wife specialists who are trained in the scientific approach and, who, in addition, practice within the medical tradition of diagnosing, prescribing and prognosing the out-come of a patient's condition. Pregnant women are expected to accept this as an aspect of childbirth. The underlying ideology is the ideology of science. The institution which cares for birth within that ideology is the medical hospital specializing in maternity cases. This setting is imbued with the spirit of rationality in attempting to improve the mea-surable success at childbirth (perinatal mortality, morbidity, baby weight, initial weight gain, incidence of brain damage etc.), by physical interventions (monitoring, testing, accelerating labour, episiotomy, for-ceps, Caesarean section, blood transfusion etc.). Pregnant women pos-sess the same ideology as the staff to a very large extent. It also includes the view that pain is alien to human experience and should not be endured but "killed" by the use of chemical drugs administered by nurses.

The experience of childbearing can be construed as a series of events which link together important aspects of relationships between a woman and other people. Conception, pregnancy and birth are linked and mirror their counterpart, contraception, the normal menstrual cycle and abortion. These events are linked to relationships with men in courtship, betrothal and marriage, as well as with men as consorts or as transitory lovers.

There is also a firm belief that society is changing or progressing so that the events and relationships surrounding childbirth are discussed. Attempts are made at improvement and several different ways of managing childbirth occur among the same generation of people from the same position in the social structure. Western industrial society is committed to monitoring the patterns of behaviour associated with a number of institutions and stages in the life cycle. We know something of the patterns of behaviour in childbearing due to this process of monitoring. For example, contraception has increased in ease and effectiveness since 1930 and there have been changes in the preferred technique especially during the 1970s. The number of women who rear at least one child alone has risen markedly in Britain. Stigmatization of divorced and unmarried mothers has declined and the economic resources of single mothers has improved leading to an increase in their number. Breast-feeding declined first among the higher status mothers between the two World Wars. Lower status women followed the trend. During the 1960s the beginning of a trend occurred back to breast-feeding. Older, high status women from the metropolitan area started it. During the 1970s the trend spread to younger, lower status and to rural mothers.

These and similar patterns of change have given rise to the belief in "fashions", in addition to the belief in rationality. People are uneasy if they think they are conforming too much to a fashion and becoming a "slave" to it. But they are also uneasy about going completely against a fashion. In giving birth a woman states something about her personal identity in the way she adopts or rejects "fashion", whilst at the same time justifying her behaviour on rational grounds.

Underlying the choices involved in asserting individuality through use of fashion and rationality are profound changes in identity and primitive feelings about birth; primitive in the sense of being undifferentiated, relatively formless and difficult to portray in words. The identity change in essentially from one in which the woman is a peer, though a disadvantaged one legally and socially, of her mate, to one in which she is further encumbered in this relationship by having to meet the intense demands of a child. She now has the relationship of mother to her child, with the moral responsibility and need to succeed as a caring and resourceful provider of nurture and love to a totally dependent being. This arouses feelings, primitive ones, about dealing in creation, life and death and gives rise to reworking through the feelings previously associated with being a growing child, maturing but dependent in turn on her mother.

The procedures of hospitalization in the industrial countries during labour and delivery have the potential for both helping and hindering the transition in identity. Likewise they have the potential to provide experiences which aid the development from primitive feelings about birth to feelings of fulfilment. But they also have the destructive potential to traumatize women and leave them with recurring bouts of terror and impoverished relationships with their husbands and children. Procedures of hospitalization have dominated childbirth in the industrialized world for several decades. First borns are now almost always born in hospitals and in many countries all babies are. When they are not, they are monitored from a hospital and if the birth becomes a problem the woman is hospitalized during labour. (A move from hospital to home during labour is virtually unknown.) For all practical purposes all obstetric difficulties and contingencies are now known and are well enough understood for effective management to succeed in reducing the mortality and morbidity rates during childbirth to a much lower level than a generation or two ago. Some hospitals are now paying attention to the experience of childbirth. Attempts are being made to ensure that traumatization does not occur and particular attention is being paid to procedures which might help the new mother–baby bond to develop and to procedures which facilitate the change in relationship between wife and husband, rather than fracture it.

Ideally the woman has developed a relationship with a man which, whilst being a basis for economic and domestic satisfaction, has the potential for providing a child with parents. Such is the widespread emphasis on intense feelings between marriage partners in western industrialized society that the couple will feel "in love" with one another. Sexual intercourse and control of contraceptive techniques will have been arranged with mutual interests in mind and in the expectation of no conflict between the woman and her man. There is, however, a tendency to deny the need, or even the ability of the woman to have orgasmic gratification comparable with the man's. Some believe that this develops after marriage is well established and argue that childbirth itself increases this ability in women. Recognition of sexuality in women in subject to "taboo" in many contexts including during birth. Essentially the woman responds to the man's activity and she does that in a passive way. Lack of sexual intercourse for several months is not generally thought to harm women or to give rise to difficulties. Birth is not looked upon as being an experience which is sexual in nature and women are not expected to experience or express sexual excitement during labour and delivery. Those who do so tend to lose the rapport with the hospital staff.

Dissolution of marriage has become easy through separation and divorce. Many women have relationships with their husbands which tend to fracture leading to physical separation and do not contain the potential for the development of parental roles within a marriage. Typically, they both have difficulty in making demands and in meeting those of others. This is often accompanied by negative feelings about adopting the family roles of spouse and parent and similar inability to establish relationships with non-kin. This has implications during pregnancy and birth for they have difficulty in relating to people in hospitals, and afterwards for they find it difficult to adjust to the demands of a child.

During the pregnancy the woman will consult her own doctor at intervals, book into a maternity hospital and will attend a maternity clinic run by either of them. The clinic advises on diet and exercise, personal health problems such as tobacco and alcohol abuse (widespread problems in this society), sexually transmitted disease and infections (frequently near epidemic proportions especially in urban areas) and carry out medical tests to establish the health of the mother and foetus and to make a prognosis concerning the delivery. Blood and urine tests, measures of blood pressure and of pelvic size relative to foetal head size are the main part of this. During the later part of pregnancy the woman will attend some educational classes arranged by a hospital or privately at which an expert, usually a midwife, will instruct her in how to deport herself during labour and delivery and how to manage a baby after it is born. This preparation for the role of patient in labour lays great emphasis on relaxation of mind and muscles so that fatigue and agitation do not occur. This emphasis is so great that they are sometimes called relaxation classes.

Women in hospital-run classes are encouraged to trust and depend on the staff and to gain a sufficient familiarity with the stages of birth and medical interventions for them to play the part of patient with passivity and lack of alarm. The teachers are very concerned not to give the slightest cause for alarm if they can help it. This can lead to an avoidance of discussion about pain as such a discussion might be counterproductive and raise anxiety. The fact that in European culture pain is now viewed as something to be removed by medical intervention, rather than endured, makes it difficult to discuss in the context of childbirth except in terms of analgesics and anaesthetics. Privately run classes are often similar to hospital classes but they sometimes adopt a modern trend of preparing women to give birth more actively and to be on guard against undue interference by the staff. In any case, birth is often preceded by attendance at classes which atunes the woman with the events which subsequently unfold in the labour ward and delivery room. Similarly, she will have prepared herself, by attendance at classes, discussion with friends and observation of others (an increasingly rare possibility as small family size and dispersal of nuclear families is common) for caring for a baby.

Women who are ambivalent about the roles of wife and mother may be very slow to recognize that they are pregnant. When they do become aware of it there is a strong tendency to deny its importance and a reluctance to do anything about it. The baby is, in a sense, not wanted and in some measure is treated as if it were not there. An important consequence is that the woman is less likely to gain the benefits of modern medicine and of preparation for the birth itself. Attendance at clinics is likely to be delayed and sporadic and prenatal classes not attended. Obstetric difficulties may be diagnosed too late or inadequately, increasing risk to the baby. The woman herself will not have learned very much about the staff role in childbirth which will make it difficult for her to adopt a suitable role *vis-à-vis* the staff during labour. In any case she is already likely to be suspicious or antagonistic towards those who have the authority of medical staff. Very young women, older but ambivalent women and those from poor and less educated families tend to have the greatest difficulty in coping with and benefiting from childbirth in hospital.

During pregnancy ritualistic gestures are made towards pregnant women. They have the effect of reducing the need for her to meet the demands of her previous role as money earner, daughter, autonomous individual and even as wife. She is expected to spend less energy on domestic chores, to eat more, to wear different clothes mainly attractive but a-sexual ones, to appear in public or at social gatherings less, to avoid driving cars (associated with potency and assertiveness) and to avoid carrying parcels or other loads etc. This general withdrawal from activity continues into the period after birth for several weeks. The woman will not usually oppose the suggestions that she, in effect, withdraw from her previous roles but she will remain sufficiently active to feel that she is expressing her personality and self in the home and neighbourhood even if she does reduce her activity somewhat. The reduction of demands is justified in terms of the prevailing ideology of rationality; a greater need for rest, for certain foods, for lack of muscular strain etc. Recognition of reduction of demands as a way of moving out of a previous status is not made overt. Covertly recognition is given to the possibility that necessity does not require such an emphasis on inactivity, as many tales are told of women from other cultures who, it is said, make no such adaptation and who, it is claimed, may be seen carrying such heavy loads as logs for fires only hours before delivery and who continue with it immediately afterwards. The move into decreased activity is related to the belief that birth is an ordeal for the mother. This belief is widely held and assumed and is emphasized to pregnant women, not by overt references but by avoidance of talking about it, encouragement such as "I'm sure you will be all right," "the staff are awfully good" and by discussion of how good pain killers are these days compared with a few generations ago.

Women who are making a successful transition into motherhood can be seen as undergoing a rite of passage along the lines described by Van Gennep (1908). They become separated from old roles, go through a limbo-like period of transition and are then incorporated into a new set of roles. Contact with medical experts affects each of these stages and hospitalization dominates the stage of transition. The separation stage is often well advanced before the birth and is completed on initiation into the hospital. She is already detached from being a daughter, childless wife, employee and is about to enter more fully into limbo by becoming a patient. Her clothes are sent away and she wears a standard gown. Her name is appended a hospital number. She is cleansed (shaved, washed and given an enema). Communication with her family and friends is monitored by the staff and severely curtailed. Instruments are attached to her to monitor the child's heart beat. Drugs are given to partially anaesthetize her. She is physically inspected mainly in the area of her genitals. She is expected to remain lying down and, at inspections, near delivery and afterwards, her legs are in straps which retain them in a raised and apart position. For much of the time she is alone. Staff all wear prescribed uniforms each of which indicates, to other staff, the role each is obliged to play. To the patient, distinctions other than between doctor and nurse, are difficult to make. At tense moments they all wear face masks. She is talked about and not to.

The woman who is having a good birth faces this situation with some excitement, a little anxiety and a sense of being on stage. The performance she expects to give, before an unknown but experienced and expert audience, is a very real ordeal, like an actor on a first night, but clouded in a sense of not being able to believe it is really happening at all. The woman's self has become disassociated and she feels she is an object to whom things are happening from which her real self is alienated. She trusts the soundness of the institution and she desires to have a baby. She responds readily to the depersonalizing cues in the hospital and looks forward to motherhood.

Some hospitals, aware that depersonalization can become mortification (part of a bad birth), have attempted to reduce the extreme nature of the initiation into childbearing. Some personal possessions are allowed (sponges, cold packs, flannels), husbands or other birth partners are allowed or even encouraged under strict supervision. In hospitals which have made most changes birth partners are seldom told to leave even if a Caesarean section is carried out. Suppositories have replaced enemas, shaving is dispensed with, a woman is never left alone, midwives are communicative about who is who, and about what is happening. In the first stage of labour the woman may walk about in the ward. These changes may reduce the likelihood that some women will lose their equanimity and panic or become actively hostile. (The accepted way of handling the former is to treat it as a hysterical bout with a slap on the cheek or buttock.) Nevertheless, control of the woman as a patient is fully in the hands of the staff. What she brings in is looked over. Unauthorized things are taken away. Her birth partner is given a hospital status with its own gown as a mark. The fact that some staff allow women some autonomy and fewer events of interference does not remove the quality of limbo from the woman, especially the more educated women. For less educated women and those whose background or position in the social structure (usually low status) has led them to approach life events, such as childbirth, as routines which other people practice on them and who expect hectoring and chivvying as the main means of social control, a reduction of arduous procedures and consultation with them can make them feel that the hospital is not very good. "They don't care in that place. They didn't even bother to shave me." "They kept asking *me* if I wanted things. Don't they know what to do? I don't think they know what they are doing in there. Got their minds on other things."

When a woman is ill prepared or ambivalent about her change in status the hospital experience can have a very different effect. She will tend to meet the depersonalizing features of initiation into the hospital not with the excitement and sense of being on stage, as other women do, but with foreboding. The staff appear as threatening to her wellbeing and to her baby, and she feels they are likely to destroy her. Already hostile and suspicious, she loses her sense of self as everything with which she is familiar has disappeared, clothes, possessions, choice of behaviour, negotiation with others, control over confidential facts and access to private parts of her body. This is mortifying to her and she can in turn become angry, withdrawn, childlike in dependence and compliance and ultimately identifies both the staff and herself as bad. Her view of herself, full of shame, is that she is bad and has done badly and she blames the hospital for this. Mortification by experience in hospital leaves the woman less able to move actively into a maternal role developed from her previous network of relationships but as a distraught, highly ambivalent mother of a baby. Hart (1977) provides a case study of a birth which took place in hospital with intense mortification.

The destructive effects of mortification are at their most intense if the baby dies at birth. The staff consider that the well-being of mother and baby is under their control and they accept responsibility as experts for what happens. A stillbirth threatens them with feelings of guilt. The way in which the staff manage their own feelings can help or hinder the woman who has failed to make the transition into motherhood through a hospital childbirth. Mechanisms of denial and withdrawal are frequently adopted by staff and can increase the mortification. Contact with the woman is reduced to the bare minimum necessary. The baby is hidden from her and she is told that the hospital will dispose of it. She is chided for being sad and told to look forward to a future pregnancy. Some hospitals, notably the Charing Cross Hospital in London, are beginning to counsel women about their reactions. The baby is seen and touched, given a name and a funeral held. The woman discusses her feelings which frequently involve fears about being a baby killer ("a walking coffin") who must keep away from other babies lest she harm them.

It is on the postnatal ward that the woman begins to be reincorporated into her network of relationships with other people. She begins to become a mother. Staff still retain control over her patterns of sleep, feeding and exercise and regulate her interaction with her baby. Initially the control which staff has over mother and baby is very great. The amount of contact between mother and baby is limited to a few minutes feeding once every four hours and the amount of discretion exercised by the mother in what she does and how she does it is negligible. Depending on fashion she will either be chivvied into bottle feeding or, more likely nowadays, breast-feeding with complementary bottle feeds. Gradually the contact and discretion increases.

The staff justify retaining control in terms of maternal exhaustion, advantages to the baby and so on. Some of the routine practices may, however, owe more to the difficulties of administering a large hospital ward. The effects are that the patient who has given birth is slowly introduced into a new status. Some hospitals have sought to return control over herself and over her baby as soon as possible to the mother. This speeds up the process.

Personal possessions begin to appear. Her own night gown and then, after a few days, her own clothes are brought to her. Messages of congratulations and tributes in the form of flowers are received from friends which reflect that she has achieved something. She is talked to and helped by the staff, and no longer talked about and told what to do. What she has achieved and what she is being helped to do is closely identified with being a wife who has entered motherhood. A special hour is set aside when only her husband and nobody else may be with her. The gifts include things which she will use when mothering her baby. Increasingly she begins to cover herself from the gaze of other people. Breast-feeding which is often done very publicly on the ward becomes a private activity. Exercises are suggested and sometimes demonstrated with the aim of helping the woman to get her figure back. Emphasis is given to future sexual activity. Discussion of this appears to be less restricted when it is with people who have just given birth which enhances the adoption of a more complete role as wife with acceptance of sexual needs. But greater emphasis is given to restoring the body to a condition so that the woman may bear another child easily. Not only are waists expected to become slender but the uterus must be helped to shrink and the pelvic floor to gain in strength ready for another pregnancy. The new identity of mother begins to carry with it the implication that the woman must be ready to adopt the role of childbearer again at some time in the future.

After about a week the mother leaves hospital and is physically reincorporated into her home with her baby. As far as the hospital is concerned they are discharged patients. Medical monitoring continues to occur. The home is visited by health visitors who are experts trained in the care of babies and mother and baby are expected to attend clinics for medical checks from time to time.

Attendance at Antenatal Classes

One of the disadvantages of giving birth in hospital is that the mother may come to feel that she is regarded by the staff, not as an individual, but as a passive object to be processed. Routinization, which economizes on decision-making and instruction-giving, is essential for the smooth functioning of a hospital. It increases the likelihood that management will be comprehensive and systematic, and in turn contributes to the sense of security of the mother. At the same time, however, it can lead to a loss of identity, and alienation.

The risk of this happening is likely to be reduced if the mother regularly attends antenatal classes. These are designed to encourage the mother to do what is within her power to improve the well-being of herself and her baby. She is warned about the harm caused by smoking during pregnancy, she is taught exercises to ease delivery and she is encouraged to breast-feed. But, quite apart from its specific benefits, the antenatal class can confer the intangible but valuable benefit of giving the mother a feeling of belonging in the hospital. By contrast with the antenatal clinic, where the mother may be seen by a different doctor each time she attends, and then rather briskly after a long wait, the antenatal class offers her the opportunity of establishing contact with the institution at a personal level. She will meet with the same instructor and the same group of mothers each week, the atmosphere will be informal, and any anxieties due to a lack of familiarity with the hospital and its procedures should diminish. The resulting improvement in her self-confidence is beneficial not only to her but also to those responsible for her management, since she is likely to be more cooperative and less demanding.

With data from just over a thousand sets of obstetric notes obtained from a London teaching hospital we were able to investigate what kind of mother was likely to take advantage of antenatal classes. Our original hypothesis was that those mothers who stood to benefit most for the reasons described above, that is, mothers who were most in need of moral support for social, cultural or medical reasons, would be most likely to be regular attenders. Mothers are supposed to go to eight classes and we classified those who went to six or more as good attenders.

Specifically and, with hindsight, rather optimistically, we hypothesized that (i) mothers not living with husband or boyfriend, (ii) mothers not British and (iii) mothers with a history of miscarriages or terminations, or high blood pressure at the time of booking, would be most in need of moral support and therefore likely to be good attenders.

For the purpose of testing these hypotheses we restricted the sample to those mothers who had no previous live births. This was necessary because mothers who already have had a successful delivery are much less likely to attend classes, whatever their background. Since poor attendance in some cases is simply due to a premature delivery, we further restricted the sample to those mothers with term pregnancies. This left us with 481 cases, 57% of which were good attenders.

The results completely contradicted our hypotheses. The proportion of good attenders among mothers not living with husband or boyfriend (henceforward "solo mothers") was only 35. Of non-British mothers, only the Irish, West Indians and Asians (from the Indian sub-continent) were present in the sample in adequate numbers for tests, and the first

TABLE I
Proportion of Good Attenders in Each Age Group

Age of mother	*% good attenders*
20 or less	18
21–25	41
26 or more	67

two of these groups had very low proportions of good attenders: 22% of the Irish, 13% of the West Indians. The percentage of Asians, 41%, was also low. In the case of the three medical conditions, the proportions were not significantly different from average.

We next investigated whether the categories above differed systematically from the rest of the sample in ways that were likely to affect class attendance. Three such factors were the age of the mother, her degree of responsibility and whether or not she was recorded as having an occupation (as opposed to being unemployed or a housewife). In principle our original hypotheses might have been correct if allowance had been made for these factors.

Age did indeed prove to be an important factor. The younger the mother, the less likely she was to attend, and the proportion of young mothers among the solo mothers, Irish and West Indians was higher than average. The figures are summarized in Tables I and II.

Table III gives the percentage of good attenders in each category, disaggregated by age group. Table III shows that if attention is confined to mature mothers (those aged 26 or more), solo mothers are actually better than average attenders. The Irish, Asians and West Indians remain worse than average, but the discrepancy is much reduced.

The responsibility of the mother was assessed using four indicators present in the obstetric notes: booking early, not smoking during pregnancy, expressing a desire to breast-feed and not having a negative attitude towards the pregnancy. These indicators were all positively

TABLE II
Percentages of Solo Mothers, Irish, Asians and West Indians in Each Age Category

Age of mother	*Solo mothers*	*Irish*	*Asians*	*West Indians*	*Whole sample*
20 or less	42	13	9	53	9
21–25	27	48	31	13	23
26 or more	31	40	59	33	68

TABLE III

Percentages of Good Attenders among Solo Mothers, Irish, Asians and West Indians, by Age Category

Age of mother	Solo mothers	Irish	Asians	West Indians	Whole sample
20 or less	0	0	33	0	18
21–25	29	9	20	0	41
26 or more	88	44	53	40	67

correlated with one another, and with good class attendance, at the 5% significance level or better, with a single exception: the association between early booking and wishing to breast-feed was only significant at the 13% level. Table IV shows the percentage of each category scoring positively on each indicator, and Table V gives the percentage of good attenders among those who scored positively.

The West Indians and Asians score well on the responsibility indicators, the solo mothers poorly and the Irish very poorly. If the sample is restricted to those scoring positively on the indicators, the percentage of good attenders among the Irish increases substantially and among the other categories slightly, but in each case they are well below average for the sample as a whole. Further restricting the sample to mature mothers (those aged 26 or more) causes a great improvement in all the figures, especially for solo mothers who now have a better-than-average percentage of good attenders. But the other three categories still remain 20–30% below average.

These results suggest that the low percentage of good attenders among the four categories may be explained as follows.

TABLE IV

Percentage of Solo Mothers, Irish, Asians and West Indians Scoring Positively on Each Responsibility Indicator

Responsibility indicator	Solo mothers	Irish	Asians	West Indians	Whole sample
booking early	54	44	81	73	72
not smoking during pregnancy	54	48	91	87	76
wishing to breast-feed	81	57	75	93	80
having a positive attitude	62	74	97	80	92

TABLE V
**Percentage of Good Attenders among Solo Mothers, Irish, Asians
and West Indians Scoring Positively on Each Responsibility
Indicator**

Responsibility indicator	Solo mothers	Irish	Asians	West Indians	Whole sample
booking early	28	30	50	18	68
not smoking during pregnancy	43	27	38	15	62
wishing to breast-feed	38	31	42	14	59
having a positive attitude	38	24	43	17	59

In the case of the solo mothers, by the high proportion of very young in that category. The older solo mothers are in fact better-than-average attenders.

The West Indians have an even higher proportion of very young mothers, but although age is certainly a factor, it does not appear to be the dominant one. The West Indians score well on the responsibility indicators, so their poor attendance figures remain largely unexplained.

The Irish have a higher-than-average proportion of young mothers and they score below average on the responsibility indicators (even when the sample is restricted to mature mothers), so these are both factors. But again these factors can be only a partial explanation because the attendance figures remain a long way below average even when the sample is restricted to mature mothers scoring positively on the indicators.

The obstetric notes included the occupation of the mother as stated at booking, no doubt subject to substantial recording error. The information was used to test the hypothesis that workers (those classified as professionals, skilled workers, unskilled workers or entrepreneurs) would have less time to attend classes than non-workers (housewives, students and the unemployed), and would have lower percentages of good attenders. In fact, their figure was 61% as opposed to 40% for non-workers. For solo mothers, the Irish, the Asians and the West Indians, the percentages of good attenders among those classified as workers were 42%, 26%, 56% and 20% respectively, in each case higher than in the unrestricted sample. This factor was accordingly discounted.

A systematic analysis disaggregating the solo mothers, Irish, Asians and West Indians by separate occupation was precluded by the small number of observations in many of the cells. Professionals, skilled workers and entrepreneurs had the highest percentages of good attenders, both for the sample as a whole and for the subsample of mature mothers. The Irish, Asians and West Indians (but not the solo mother) had below average percentages in these occupations but this was not necessarily even a partial explanation of their low percentages of good attenders. To clarify the issue, further disaggregation by age would have been required and this was not worthwhile given the small sizes of the subsamples.

One is left with the conclusion that those who would benefit most from the general support provided by antenatal classes tend to attend least; the solo mothers, because they tend to be young; the Irish, Asians and West Indians, probably mainly for cultural reasons, perhaps because they feel (or think that they would feel) out of place. For the Irish and West Indians, youth is also a factor. And in the case of the Irish, the poor showing on the responsibility indicators appears to be a further partial explanation.

One of the aims of antenatal classes is to encourage breast-feeding. Breastmilk is nutritionally superior to infant formula and, probably more important still, confers a protection against ill-health which is particularly useful in the first three months of life.

In the sample, the proportion of mothers who were breast-feeding on discharge was very high, regardless of whether or not they had attended antenatal classes, but good attenders were more likely to breast-feed than poor attenders, 97% as opposed to 85%.

Fairly obviously, these figures do not warrant the conclusion that classes are successful in this particular objective, for it can (and should) be argued that those mothers who are good attenders tend to be informed and responsible, and therefore likely to include a high percentage of breast-feeders in any case. This is confirmed when one checks on the intentions of the mother with regard to feeding recorded at booking. Ninety-eight per cent of those who were breast-feeding at discharge said that they would do so at booking. The association between feeding intentions and outcome was significant at the 1% level, and the association between feeding intentions and good class attend-

TABLE VI
Percentage Breast-feeding at Discharge, by Class Attendance

	Poor	Good
Of those intending to breast-feed	91	99
Of those not intending to breast-feed	21	40

ance was significant at the 3% level. It is therefore not surprising that the association between feeding outcome and good class attendance was significant at the 1% level.

To evaluate the influence of classes one must therefore look at the outcome holding intentions constant. Table VI shows that backsliders (those who said they would breast-feed, but did not) were more common among poor class attenders than good ones, and improvers (those who said they would not, but did) were less common among poor attenders than good ones.

This, of course, does not end the story. There are strong associations between tendency to breast-feed and marital status, country of origin, age, the responsibility indicators, and occupation, each being significant

TABLE VII

Percentage Breast-feeding at Discharge, by Class Attendance and Other Factors

	Poor	Good
Marital status		
mother living with husband or boyfriend	88	96
solo mother	67	100
Country of origin		
U.K.	82	97
Ireland	58	67
Asia	93	100
West Indies	90	100
Age		
20 or less	71	67
21–25	82	95
26 or more	93	98
Responsibility indicators		
booked early	86	97
booked late	82	96
did not smoke during pregnancy	89	97
smoked	75	94
had a positive attitude	86	96
had a negative attitude	60	100
Occupation		
professional	100	99
entrepreneur	100	100
skilled	87	98
unskilled	68	70
unemployed	60	100
housewife	81	94
student	90	100

at the 5% level or better. Since all of these had a significant association with class attendance, each could in principle be held to account for the association between class attendance and breast-feeding. It was therefore necessary to investigate each of these factors on the same lines as feeding intentions. The results are presented together in Table VII.

It can be seen that in each case, in each subcategory, good class attenders are more likely to breast-feed than poor ones (with one exception, very young mothers). The biggest differences were among solo mothers and those who scored negatively on the responsibility indicators.

Looking at the columns in Table VII separately, one may generalize the analysis of the determinants of breast-feeding holding constant the influence of class attendance. It can be seen that the Irish, the very young and the unskilled stand out as being least likely to breast-feed, regardless of class attendance; more detailed analysis shows that, although these categories overlap to some extent, these conclusions remain valid independently.

References

Chard, T. and Richards, M. (1977). *Benefits and Hazards of the New Obstetrics*. London: Heinemann.

Dick-Read, G. (1933). *Childbirth without Fear*. London: Heinemann. (1968 edition).

Donnison, J. (1977). *Midwives and Medical Man*. London: Heinemann.

Hart, N. (1977). "Parenthood and Patienthood". In *Medical Encounters* (A. Davis and G. Horobin, eds). London: Croom Helm.

Kitzinger, S. and Davis, J. A. (1978). *The Place of Birth*. Oxford: Oxford University Press.

Lamaze, F. (1958). *Painless Childbirth*. London: Burke.

Leboyer, F. (1975). *Birth without Violence*. London: Wildwood House.

Menzies, I. (1960). "A Case Study in the Function of Social Systems as a Defence against Anxiety". *Human Relations* **13**, (2).

Van Gennep, A. (1908). *The Rites of Passage*. London: Routledge. (1960 edition; English translation).

Velvovsky, I. Z. (1972). "Psychoprophylaxis in Obstetrics: A Soviet Method". In *Modern Perspectives in Psycho-obstetrics* (J. G. Howells, ed.). Edinburgh: Oliver and Boyd.

Index